T0157085

SURVIVAL GUIDE

═══ FOR THE ═══

DENTAL PATIENT

*How to Pick the Best
Dentist, Save Money, and
Protect Your Health*

ALEXANDER CORSAIR, D.M.D.

iUniverse, Inc.
Bloomington

Survival Guide for the Dental Patient
How to Pick the Best Dentist, Save Money, and Protect Your Health

iUniverse books may be ordered through booksellers or by contacting:

iUniverse
1663 Liberty Drive
Bloomington, IN 47403
www.iuniverse.com
1-800-Authors (1-800-288-4677)

ISBN: 978-1-4697-4702-6 (sc)
ISBN: 978-1-4697-4701-9 (hc)
ISBN: 978-1-4697-4700-2 (e)

Library of Congress Control Number: 2012901030

Printed in the United States of America

iUniverse rev. date: 3/1/2012

I would like to thank my wife, Phyllis Corsair, for the hours she spent proofreading and editing the manuscript. Without her help and patience this project would not have been possible.

Contents

INTRODUCTION

While treating dental patients for 45 years I've observed types of behavior that enabled good outcomes and other behavior that contributed to dental disasters. The actions you take to prevent or treat dental problems are a result of your attitudes, experiences, knowledge and to some extent financial resources. **The information contained in this guide will help you choose better dentists, save money, and achieve better dental health.**

Are you likely to have a major dental problem in the future? If you are a smoker, a diabetic or have a family history of gum disease then you are at higher risk for future dental problems.

Thirty-four thousand new cases of cancer of the oral cavity are diagnosed annually.[1] If you use tobacco and alcohol your risk for developing oral cancer is increased thirty- seven fold.

Twenty-five percent of Americans over the age of 65 have lost all of their teeth.[2] Obviously these patients made bad choices. The complete removable denture is a failure because it is uncomfortable and it impairs speech and eating. Wearing a full denture is also depressing since it has traditionally symbolized old age and infirmity. The denture has a negative impact on speech and social intercourse generally.

In 2010, $108,000,000,000 that is one hundred and eight billion dollars was spent for dental services in the United States. How much money would you like to contribute next year?

You will find information in this guide to help you reduce dental expenses

---

1   www.AmericanCancerSociety.org
2   Centers for Disease Control and Prevention. Tooth loss among persons greater than 65 years old. M.M.W.R. 48;296 1999

and have more pleasant dental experiences. Many patients find the dental experience painful and frightening.

The information in this book will show you how to find a dentist to provide a pain free experience. As a dentist and teacher since 1967 I have interacted with many hundreds of general dentists and specialists. They have different interests and personalities. As you read through this book you will learn how to identify the type of dentist that suits your needs. The information you will find in this book will help you identify your needs as a dental patient. You will also learn the facts about how your health can be affected by dental disease and how your general health can affect your dental health.

I have served as an expert witness in dental malpractice cases since 1982.

Included in this book is information to help you decide how to deal with unsatisfactory dental treatment. Do you feel you have been mistreated? What are your options?

Since 1971 I have been a practicing periodontist and educator. While the specifics of the book are about dental care, many of these basic principles apply to being a successful medical patient as well. These principles apply to getting the best service from any professional.

CHAPTER 1	Prevention of Dental Disease: Nine Ways to Save Your Money and Your Health

It is well known that good dental health will enhance your chewing, speech and esthetics and prevent the dreaded "toothache". It is said that people who smile often live longer.

Recently it has been shown that oral inflammation may contribute to systemic diseases especially to a higher incidence of fatal heart attack and stroke.[3]

So it's not just "Be true to your teeth or they will be false to you". If your mouth is not healthy your risk of acquiring a systemic disease is greater. It has been said that oral inflammation is a greater risk factor for heart attack than high cholesterol. Much has already been written about prevention of dental disease and information is available on the internet from organizations such as the American Dental Association and the American Academy of Periodontology. See the appendix for their web sites. The following behaviors will help to minimize dental disease:

1. Maintain a diet with a low frequency of retentive (sticky) carbohydrates. A low frequency means once or twice a day.

---

3   Ridker PM, Silvertown JD. Inflamation, C-Reactive Protein and Atherothrombosis. Journal of Periodontology Supplement Workshop on Inflamation 2008;79:1544-1551

2. Brush and floss at least once a day. Flossing must be done every day, not occasionally, to prevent gingivitis.

Have your dentist or his hygienist teach you the proper technique. I've seen some horrible approaches to flossing. For example, using the floss forward and back like a saw. Ouch!

The proper technique involves holding a small segment of floss between the thumb and index finger of each hand and slowly sliding the floss between 2 adjacent teeth. Slide the floss under the gum and then press the floss laterally against the tooth then slide the floss toward the chewing surface of the tooth. Do this for each tooth surface. Use lightly waxed floss. With experience, flossing takes about 5 minutes to complete. Figures 1 & 2 below illustrate how to hold and place dental floss. At first your gums will bleed in many areas but after flossing daily, the bleeding will stop because the inner lining of the gum will have healed. Healing occurs because the floss, used properly, will remove sticky bacteria from below the gum line. Tooth brushing alone will not do this. The water pick will not remove attached bacterial plaque. You should have your dentist demonstrate the technique. Then have the dentist watch as you floss under his or her supervision.

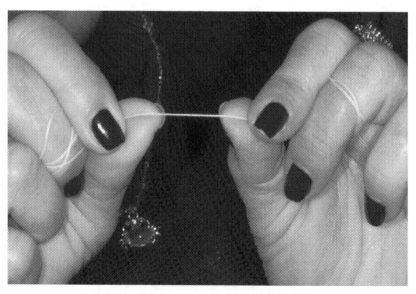

Figure 1. Proper technique for holding floss

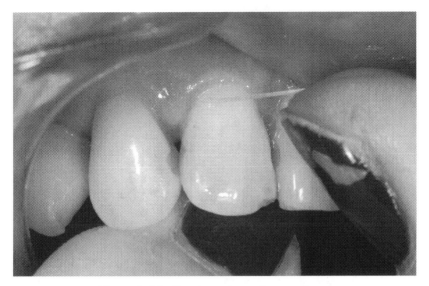

Figure 2. Use floss between and around teeth

3. See your dentist 2 to 4 times a year for an examination of your teeth, gums and oral mucosa.

Have the dentist do an oral cancer exam. Thirty-four thousand Americans are diagnosed with oral cancer each year. The cure rate is only 50%. If you smoke and drink alcohol regularly your risk is increased 37 times.[4] At these visits X-rays may be taken and a cleaning should be done. Every 3 to 5 years a complete set of X-rays (18 films) should be taken. This is necessary to visualize the bone above the teeth to check for bone loss and other pathology such as cysts and tumors.

4. If you are a periodontal patient or might become one (family history of periodontal disease, diabetes, and smoking are risk factors) then you should have cleanings and exams every 3 months. A periodontal sensitivity test is available. It shows if you have the gene that predisposes a person to periodontal disease. You should alternate exams and cleanings between a periodontist and your general dentist even if one of the hygienists says, "Oh you can just come here for all of your cleanings." That might be good for her but not for you! It's best to alternate visits for cleanings.

4   www.American Cancer Society.org

5. Use an over the counter fluoride mouthwash if you are decay prone. ACT is one such rinse.

As we age salivary production decreases and the resultant dry mouth is more prone to significant decay. Water fluoridation has reduced decay by 25 %. In spite of the obvious effectiveness of water fluoridation, only 27 states have fluoridated drinking water. An additional 50% reduction in decay can be achieved by having sealants placed on a child's molars. Sealants can be applied by the general dentist as soon as the permanent molars are present. This is a very cost effective procedure. Typically children who develop large cavities become adults who need caps, bridges, root canals and possibly dental implants.

If you are a periodontal patient not under good control, ask about a Chlorhexidiene rinse (Peridex). A Chlorhexidiene rinse will reduce the number of bacteria in the mouth by 60%. It will stain the teeth if your plaque control isn't excellent. The stain can be removed by the dentist.

Prescriptions for the rinse are covered by drug plans. This is a good investment even if not covered, especially if you have had recurrent gingivitis. A generic is now available. Listerine is less effective than Peridex but it does not stain teeth. It must be used 4 times per day to be effective.

Also ask about Periostat which is a low dose Doxycycline tablet. Periostat is helpful if you are a smoker. Periostat modulates the over response to plaque that some periodontal patients express. Unfortunately it only helps 30 % of patients using it. I have not seen any adverse effects. It is covered by prescription drug plans. Consider, if your disease is severe, having cleanings every 2 months. One study showed that patients having cleanings done every 2 weeks over a 2-year period had perfectly controlled periodontal disease and no decay. This frequency is not practical but makes a good point about the impact of professional cleanings.

6. Smoking is a major causative factor for periodontal disease. A periodontal problem will never be fully controlled if the patient smokes. Get help and quit smoking. There are several medications available by prescription which

can help with nicotine withdrawal symptoms. Consult with your physician or dentist regarding the use of these drugs.

7. Diabetes is a causative factor for periodontal disease and it is also true that your diabetes will not be well controlled if you have active periodontal disease.[5] If you don't get your diabetes under control, you will have poorly controlled periodontal disease. A very well controlled diabetic should have glycated hemoglobin (A1C) of less than 7%.

8. Clenching and grinding your teeth, known as bruxism, will contribute to periodontal disease, broken fillings and TMJ problems. Have a hard acrylic upper night guard made. It will protect your teeth from chipping. It will also prevent teeth from becoming loose due to grinding and clenching.

9. Find a good dentist. Select one who is appropriate for you.
   How do you do that? The process is described later in the book.

To summarize, good oral hygiene (brushing and flossing every day) and professional care at least twice a year has been proven to be a powerful tool to control and prevent dental disease.

If you have children, have them see the dentist for topical fluorides, sealants and oral hygiene instruction. Substitute fruits and raw vegetables for sugar containing snacks. Regularly scheduled dental visits are not simply a way for dentists to make more money. Purchasing expensive dental treatment like caps and implants and then not bothering to have twice a year professional care is self destructive behavior. I have seen so many patients self destruct. Typically, 4 years after the completion of treatment the patients who have had no professional preventive care regress back to their original level of disease. This poor response to treatment without professional maintenance has been reported in studies in the Journal of Periodontology. Regular exams give the dentist an opportunity to find small areas of decay. Waiting until it hurts results in more extensive and expensive treatment. Large areas of decay

---

5   Taylor GW, Bidirectional Interrelation between Diabetes & Periodontal Disease. Annals of Periodontology Dec 2001;6:880

can not be restored with fillings. When very little tooth structure remains the tooth will need to be restored with a cap or crown as it is called in the profession. Persistent pain from a tooth often means root canal treatment is required. The Endodontist or root canal specialist needs to open a large hole in the middle of the tooth to gain access to remove the dead nerve. Following endodontic treatment a cap or crown is usually required. Establish good dental habits for your children. The money they will save as adults can be used to buy a house or at least a new car.

CHAPTER 2 | | First Step, Finding the
Best Dentist for You

How do you find the best dentist for you? You may have a friend that loves his dentist.

However your friend may have different needs as a dental patient.

I want you to sit down and make a list of the things you didn't like about your previous dentist. Now make a list, in order of importance, of the things you would appreciate in a new dentist. The list should include things like gender, age, location, available parking, the dentist's personality, commitment to quality and comprehensive care, fee scale, availability of modern techniques, the size of the practice (multi doctor with large staff v. solo doctor with small staff). Does the practice have evening hours and Saturday hours? Are the dentists preferred providers in an insurance network in which you are insured? For example, if you do not have dental insurance you might be better off in a practice that is not an insurance practice. You should get more personalized treatment in this type of fee for service practice.

Another source of referral to a general dentist is the local periodontist. A periodontist will usually refer to a dentist who also refers to him or her, but since many general dentists refer to the periodontist, he or she will refer you to one of the better general dentists in the area. When the same name comes up more than once, you then have verification.

So "To thine own self be true". If you are a frightened dental patient then by all means find a dentist who specializes in apprehensive patients. This means more than just saying "We cater to cowards". There are general dentists who are certified dental anesthesiologists. Intravenous sedation may or may not be appropriate for you and it will add to the cost of treatment. See a dentist who provides some type of sedation. The dentist must have a certificate issued by the state to provide sedation. At the minimum see a dentist who provides nitrous oxide analgesia (sweet air). Sweet air is safe for all patients regardless of their medical history. The effects of sweet air wear off in less than 5 minutes. There are no after effects so you may drive afterwards. Sweet air creates mild euphoria and moderate analgesia. The effect of sweet air is similar to drinking 8 ounces of alcohol. Most patients like feeling inebriated but some patients don't like feeling a loss of control. In any event sweet air is a pleasant experience and you will still be aware of what is going on. You will still require good local anesthesia to prevent pain. Sweet air is adequate to relieve mild to moderate apprehension but is not adequate for the very apprehensive patient who will respond better to I.V. sedation. All oral surgeons are trained to use I.V. sedation. The oral surgeons' training includes almost a year of anesthesia training. Some general dentists receive training after dental school in the use of sedation. It is difficult to determine how well trained they are. Of course a dentist with training as a dental anesthesiologist will have been trained in all forms of anesthesia and sedation as well as being trained in how to handle complications.

If you are a frightened patient who should you choose? It depends on how frightened you are and your medical history. If you require general dentistry, are very frightened and you have many medical issues then use a general dentist certified in anesthesiology. Very few periodontists are trained to use I.V. sedation. If the periodontist you have chosen is not trained to use sedation you may ask him to use a dental anesthesiologist to provide sedation during your implant surgery or during your periodontal surgery. Usually the surgery can be done in one visit. This will help with the cost of the sedation since multiple visits will cost more than one long visit

Verify that the dentist is comfortable with these aids and does not merely tolerate apprehensive patients. This attitude must be true with your other requirements as well.

You may call the local dental society, a local dental school or a local hospital to obtain a recommendation for the type of dentist you need. Call a hospital with a dental residency program. Hospital residency programs and dental schools will have attending dentists who are trained in sedation. Get several names if possible. At that point you should check the internet to see if these dentists have websites. While it is true that the web site will depict the practice in the best possible light, it will explain the available services and the essence of the practice as well as the dentist's credentials.

What are good credentials? Examples of good credentials are: an appointment to a dental school as an assistant professor or higher rank, fellowships in an academy like the Academy of General Dentistry or the American College of Dentists, hospital appointments, and papers published in dental journals, and years of practice experience with few or no disciplinary problems. The state education department has records of disciplinary actions taken against dentists. The health department keeps records of disciplinary actions against physicians.

I would not suggest selecting a relative or close friend to be your dentist. It is difficult for a friend or relative to be objective while making a diagnosis and preparing a treatment plan. Dealing with payment is also awkward. In some cases a dentist who is also a relative may not charge you for dental treatment. What do you do if you are not happy with the results of treatment? It can also be difficult for the dentist who must do an unpleasant procedure for a relative especially a wife, or his child. My observation is that the patient with a relative as a dentist is usually under treated because the dentist is trying to be "too kind" to the patient. The best choice is to pick an unrelated dentist.

Who is the best dentist for your child? Pediatric dentistry is a specialty. Some pediatric dentists are also trained to do orthodontics. I believe that children should be treated by pediatric dentists since they are specifically trained to treat children. Obviously they also enjoy treating children. The child's experience will generally be more pleasant especially if the child is apprehensive. The pediatric dentist is trained to help children who are frightened.

| CHAPTER 3 | | Your First Visit with the New Dentist. How to Communicate Effectively |

Now, armed with a short list in order of preference, make a preliminary phone call.

Tell the receptionist that you are a prospective new patient and you have several questions to ask about the practice. Ask if the office manager would call you back when she has time to speak to you for a few minutes. When this individual calls back you will ask about the things that are important to you. For example if this information was not available on the web site: what is the office schedule? Do they have reserved parking for patients? Do they have handicap access? You may ask about the doctors' training and ask if an office brochure can be sent to you. You may also want to ask about the number of staff members employed in the practice.

What insurance plans do they participate in? Never ask if they "accept your insurance". Accept is a vague term. You really need to know if the doctor is a preferred provider in your plan and accepts the fee schedule stipulated by the plan. A dentist may not participate in your plan or any plan in fact but he or she may routinely submit a pre determination of benefits and then accept as partial payment those benefits leaving you to pay only the balance.

Note how patient the office manager is with your questions. She usually represents the personality of the doctor and the practice. Follow this routine with 2 or 3 phone calls and then decide which practice to call to set up an appointment. When you do this, ask what will be done on the first visit, what payment will be expected, how it may be paid and how long the appointment will be. What you should expect, in a quality office, is a pleasant greeting almost immediately upon your arrival. You should be asked to fill out a complete medical and dental history and the usual financial and insurance information. You should then get to meet the dentist who should review your history and ask how they can help you. At that point you need to tell the dentist about all of your concerns. Show the dentist a wish list for your dental future.

This information is confidential so there is no need to hold anything back.

I have had patients fail to tell me about medications; fail to tell me that they usually faint with dental injections, etc. Withholding information can be hazardous to your health. I have declined to treat patients who have done this. Trust goes both ways. Avoid being critical of your previous dentist or dentists. If you have had bad experiences, simply state the facts as you recall them. Blaming your existing dental problems on your previous dentist does not score points with the new dentist. It simply makes the new dentist feel that you are a complainer and he will be next on your list of "bad" dentists. In fact this type of behavior, if extreme, may motivate the new dentist to decline to accept you into the practice. There is no obligation to accept you as a patient. "I'm sorry but I don't think I'm going to be able to solve your problems and satisfy your needs".

Given that you are satisfied with the practice you will typically return after the first visit for a consultation .On the first visit the dentist will have collected data from his exam and will have obtained X -rays and possibly study models and photographs. A complete set of X-rays often consists of 18 films. This is what is required to see all areas of the mouth and all of the teeth. You may have seen a panoramic X-ray unit. Typically this machine circles your head and in 10 seconds captures all of the structures from your nose to below your chin. This type of X-ray gives the dentist a broad view but not the detail provided by peri apical intra oral films.

Radiation exposure is not an issue today with sensitive film that requires less radiation. Of course you will wear a lead apron during the X-ray procedure.

New patients often complain that they are afraid of too much radiation. This same person will spend hours in the sun absorbing much more radiation than the dental X-rays deliver. A Full series of X-rays should only be taken every 3 to 5 years.

A newer diagnostic tool found in some dental offices today is the Cone Beam CT Scan.

This devise captures axial images of one or both jaws. The computer program then reformats the captured data into several different images. These images include a panoramic view, an axial view, a cross sectional view and a 3d model view. Originally CT scans were used by oral surgeons and periodontists to plan implant cases. Patients were referred to radiologists for this service. The fee for the CT scan, $350 to $500, was paid for by the patient's medical insurance but today that is rarely the case. With the advent of small cone beam ct scanners, some dentists have CBCT scanners in their offices. Most of the dentists having CBCT scanners are oral surgeons or periodontists. However more recently Orthodontists and Endodontist have found these scanners useful in their diagnosis and treatment planning. Several newspaper articles as well as articles in dental journals have criticized dentists for the over usage of scanners as merely a way to make more money.[6] The truth is that for some procedures this technology is very helpful.

For example, when planning multiple implants the scan is the best way to see the available volume of bone. It is also the most accurate way to measure the distance from vital structures such as major nerves in the lower jaw and sinuses in the upper jaw.

On the other hand cases with an abundance of bone or cases with one implant can often be done without a scan. In orthodontics as well, some cases can be better evaluated with a scan.

Radiation is a minor factor with CBCT whereas medical CT scans had more radiation.

In any event, at the second visit the dentist should present a plan of treatment and possibly alternative plans. He should also include the fees for treatment and the time line for completing the treatment planned. Certainly

---

6   N.Y. TIMES, 11/22/10, "Radiation worries for children in the Dentists chair."

you should come to this visit with your significant other. Indicate, after the dentist has answered all of your questions that you would like a copy of the treatment plan and you would like to think about the plan. Thank the dentist for his time What ever fee charged for this examination and consultation is usually small compared to the time spent by the dentist and his staff. You might ask if the fee will be credited to your future treatment.

If you picked the dentist carefully, then you probably will be satisfied with the plan.

You may have been told that the treatment would be done in stages. In some cases this is not possible. If you are having upper and lower teeth capped, the dentist will need to do both the upper and lower at the same time. If you are having several implants done in the upper then all of the implants are done at the same time. In this way the implants can be better angled and spaced. It is also easier for the patient, in most cases, to have one longer visit rather than several surgical visits, each of them requiring antibiotics, ice and pain medications.

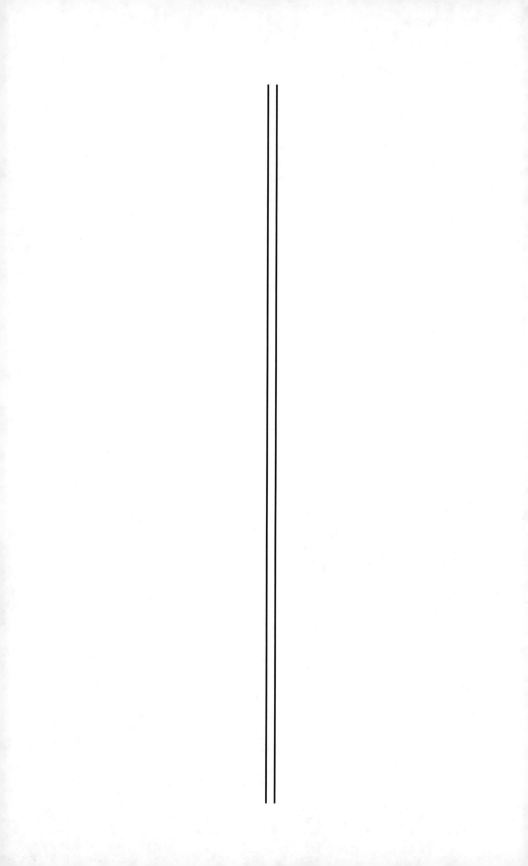

CHAPTER 4   How to Have Pain Free
                                                Dental Visits

The key to having a pain free experience is to discuss pain control with the dentist well in advance of having any dental surgery. Clearly and politely state your needs. The dentist will describe the available options. Most dental procedures are surgical. The dentist, depending on the procedure, is cutting tooth structure, gum tissue or bone. Of course some type of anesthesia is required. Many years ago while serving as a dental officer in the Navy I had an opportunity to treat a rugged old Marine sergeant. As I prepared to administer a local anesthetic the Marine said, "Hey doc I don't need that, I can take the pain". I politely replied, "I'm sure you can but I can't". It's difficult for most dentists to do precise high quality work knowing that the patient is feeling pain.

The type of anesthesia depends on the procedure, the patient and the patients' response to dental care. The following things can be done to help eliminate pain:

1. Have local anesthesia for all procedures

2. Have a topical anesthetic gel applied before the injection.

3. If you are an apprehensive patient, ask the dentist to use sweet air or nitrous oxide before the dental injection and during the entire procedure. It is safe and effective. There are no contra indications to the use of nitrous oxide. The effects wear off immediately so that you may drive afterwards. On the other hand some patients don't like the feeling of losing some control.

4. Ask the dentist if you may wear head phones and listen to your favorite music. Make the music loud enough so you can not hear the sound of the drill.

5. In some cases it may be helpful to take Vicodin or some other narcotic analgesic medication 30 minutes before the visit. Discuss this with the dentist.

6. Some dentists may prescribe a drug like Valium before the visit. This drug in conjunction with nitrous oxide will provide a sedative effect as well as an analgesic (pain reduction) effect.

7. **Finally do not move when the dentist is operating. By move I mean do not close your mouth or turn your face away from the dentist unexpectedly. If you do this the dentist may accidently injure your lip, tongue or other area of your mouth which is not numb. If you need to close your mouth or scratch your nose, have a predetermined signal so the dentist will stop working.** I have had many patients fold their lower lip over their lower teeth while having these teeth cleaned. This is an attempt to protect sensitive teeth and it's a bad idea. Instead ask the dentist to numb the teeth. This is a better idea and is better for the health of your lower lip. I have had patients continually close their mouths making it necessary for me to say "Open please" dozens of times during the procedure. This is distracting to the dentist and may be harmful to the patient if the lower lip closes on a surgical instrument. **If you can't keep your mouth open, ask the dentist to use a rubber mouth prop. This is a small rubber wedge that is placed between the back teeth allowing you to relax your muscles and still have your mouth open.**

8. A select group of patients are so apprehensive that they require I.V. sedation. This is for the patient who can not tolerate pressure even without pain. This patient does not want to be aware of the procedure. Who might best provide this service was discussed earlier in the chapter on selecting the best dentist for you.

To summarize, apprehensive patients or patients with a dental phobia can have comfortable and successful dental experiences. The key is to select a dentist who is comfortable and competent with the apprehensive dental patient. With the dentist's advice choose a safe and effective modality to allay your fears, enable you to be a cooperative patient and allow the dentist to provide a high quality service.

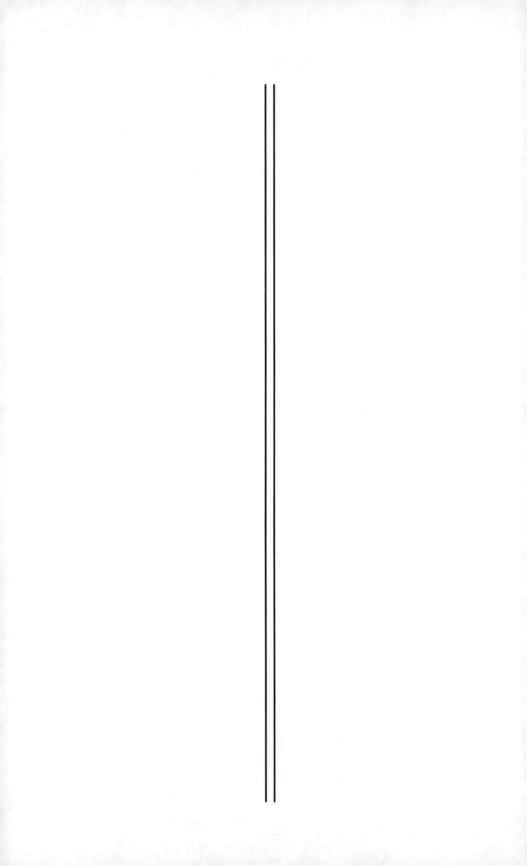

| CHAPTER 5 | How to Avoid Medical Problems in the Dental Office |

Delivering dental care often involves administration or prescription of drugs. It also involves surgery. These procedures may exacerbate medical problems.

The following is a list of things to do to avoid problems. Advise the dentist of:

1. Medical issues and drugs that you take.

2. Allergies that you have, such as to penicillin, latex or any medication.

3. A history of fainting in a dental office.

4. A history of prolonged bleeding after extraction of a tooth or after dental surgery.

5. A phobia to dental procedures.

6. All surgery you have had such as placement of a joint prosthesis, an artificial heart valve, a pacemaker, an organ transplant or heart surgery.

Ask the dentist what type of sterilization is used. Instruments contaminated with blood and not properly sterilized can transmit hepatitis B and or C. Most dental offices are expert in proper sterile technique. Ask the dentist if the staff is trained in CPR. After January 2012 all dental facilities must be equipped with defibrillators or AED's.

People who have had heart valves replaced with pig valves or mechanical valves require premedication with Amoxicillin before dental visits. This means taking four 500 mg tablets one hour before the visit. Patients allergic to Amoxicillin are prescribed Clindamycin. Years ago people with various types of heart murmurs and mitral valve prolapse were premedicated. The American Heart Association has determined that this is no longer indicated. Premedication is now reserved for people with replaced heart valves and people with a history of endocarditis. In patients with a pig valve or artificial valve, failure to premedicate may result in infection of the valve leading to endocarditis, stroke and death. Individuals with joint replacements, a total hip prosthesis for example, are also premedicated. Failure to premedicate may result in infection of the joint prosthesis. If in doubt ask your orthopedist. Prescriptions for penicillin are commonly prescribed. Be sure to advise the dentist of any history of allergy to penicillin. An upset stomach or diarrhea is not an allergic reaction. Allergy is manifested by a rash or hives followed by difficulty with breathing. This can be a life threatening emergency. If you are a very allergic person it is a good idea to carry Epi pen, a devise used to inject epinephrine under your skin in an emergency.

Another patient requiring special management is one taking anti coagulants like Coumadin. Typically the dentist will need to know the patient's INR. The INR test result is a measure of how quickly blood coagulates. If the INR is above 3.5 then a serious issue with blood loss may occur after multiple extractions or multiple implant placements or any extensive surgical procedure. Typically the Coumadin dose will be reduced or the surgical procedure modified to prevent a serious medical problem. Patients taking 325 mg of aspirin or Plavix may have bleeding problems after surgery unless the dentist is made aware of the use of these drugs.

Patients with heart irregularities may have internal pacemakers or defibrillators. It is usually prudent not to use an ultrasonic devise to clean the patient's teeth since there is a risk to the function of the pacemaker or defibrillator. Dentists frequently use local anesthetics with epinephrine, commonly called adrenalin. This drug is safe for most patients but the amount needs to be minimized for patients with a history of heart beat irregularity (fibrillation) and also for patients taking certain blood pressure medications like Metapolol a non selective beta blocker. When in doubt, check with your physician.

The apprehensive patient who often faints after a dental injection is at risk since fainting can progress to shock and death if not treated immediately. Usually a person faints, falls to the floor and then recovers since lying on the floor allows the blood to recirculate to the brain. However, if you are unattended in a dental chair and faint, you may not recover. Of course a patient should not be left unattended. Fainting can be avoided by advising the dentist of your history. The dentist may give you oxygen and place you in a reclined position with your head lower than your heart while administering a dental injection. It will be impossible for you to faint in this position.

Verify that the dentist and his staff use the most effective sterilization techniques. The best technique for sterilizing instruments used in the mouth is the autoclave. This is steam under pressure. This devise kills 100% of all micro organisms. Other effective techniques are dry heat and the chem-clave. When doing implant surgery both my assistant and I wear sterile gloves and gowns. All surfaces that we may touch are covered with sterile drapes. This includes light handles, the dental chair and counter tops. We also use sterile water to irrigate the implant site. Sterile technique as used in a hospital operating room isn't possible in a dental office but an aseptic technique is appropriate. These techniques of sterility and asepsis are used to protect the patient and the dentist from common infections, AIDS and Hepatitis B and C. Dentistry has an excellent record of preventing disease transmission.

Finally, I suggest a medical consultation before starting extensive dental treatment for patients who have medical issues. If you take many medications have your physician give you a list of the medications. Carry this list with you so that other health care providers can make reference to it especially in an emergency. Have your physician give you a note regarding any medical issues that the dentist must be aware of and any suggested modifications in treatment.

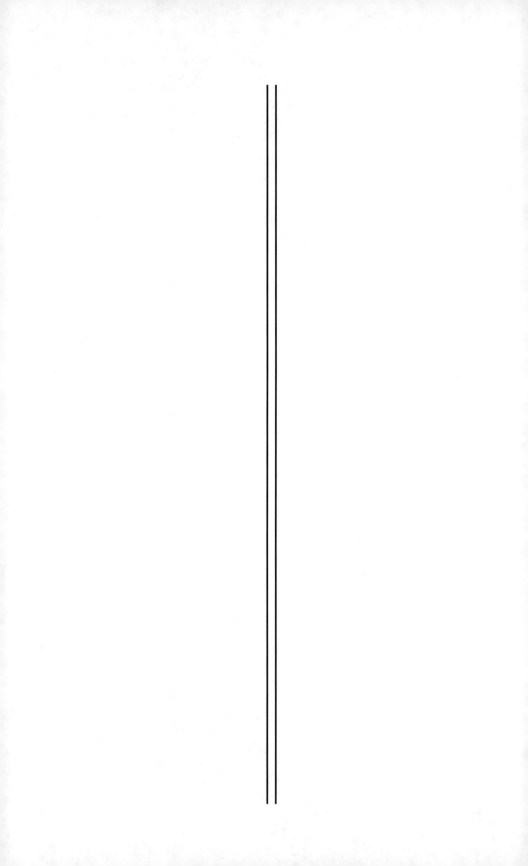

CHAPTER 6

When it's Necessary to get Other Opinions

There are many situations where a second opinion is appropriate. This may be worthwhile if you have just seen a new dentist who recommends extensive and expensive treatment. For example, the new dentist has prescribed removing all of your old restorations and replacing them with new restorations. He feels that they not of acceptable quality. He may also feel that amalgam or silver fillings are unhealthy. Is that true? Not usually. Another scenario is a recommendation that many teeth be extracted, but you feel that they are functioning normally and you have no pain. Certainly when you are told that the fee for the treatment recommended is many thousands of dollars, then you will want to consider a second opinion.

In most situations the recommendations will be valid. However some of the recommendations may be optional. Before getting another opinion ask the dentist if some of the recommendations are optional and if some treatment can wait? Also ask the dentist if there are other options that he can recommend. Then simply tell the dentist that you appreciate his or her thoroughness but you would like to get another opinion because of the extent of the required treatment.

Ask for a written treatment plan including the fees and a copy of your records including X-rays, models and any other materials that another dentist might require. You are not entitled to the original X-rays but you are entitled to a good copy. Many dentists now use digital X-rays which can be e mailed to other dentists. This is better than a hard copy. Tell the dentist that you may return for treatment but you would feel more comfortable getting another opinion.

Sometimes you may want a second opinion even when you have been treated by a dentist for many years. What do you do when teeth that were recently treated with fillings or crowns require retreatment? You should ask the dentist "why do I often break my fillings?"

Do not ask the dentist "why do your fillings always break?" Certainly don't put it that way if you plan to continue as a patient of that dentist. **Remember that beneath the gown, mask and eyewear, there is a person with feelings just like you. Not all people are dentists but all dentists are people.** You need to take responsibility, certainly until you discover why the dental restorations have failed. Often times a patient clenches or grinds their teeth and this will lead to failure even of the best work. If this is the case, ask the dentist if an appliance like a night guard will help. It usually does help and for many patients it will also prevent other problems like increased looseness or mobility of teeth and TMJ or myofacial pain.

A custom night guard appliance made by the dentist will cost between $400 and $600.

I've seen appliances in drug stores for $25 but they are large, uncomfortable and of poor quality.

I tried one myself as a learning experience. I couldn't wear it. You also need to make the "store bought" appliance your self. I will bet that I can make one better than you can and I couldn't make one that was acceptable. Spend the money. It will save you many times the cost and lots of time at the dentist in the future. Of course you will need to wear it.

If you feel that you might be uncomfortable wearing an appliance that covers all of your teeth then speak to your dentist about smaller appliances. Appliances can be made to cover only the upper front teeth and I wear one that covers only my 2 upper front teeth. How long do they last? About five years.

If you feel that your dentists' work isn't holding up long enough you may want to get another opinion. Get a complete written estimate of the new work that is proposed as well as a copy of your X-rays and take them to another dentist. Choose a dentist as I outlined in chapter 2. Tell your current dentist that you value his opinion but that you will be more comfortable getting another opinion. A health care professional should never be insulted or angry when an existing patient wants another opinion.

When you see the new dentist he may tell you that the restorative dentistry previously done was a heroic effort by your dentist to restore teeth in a simple and inexpensive way with simple fillings rather than caps or crowns. You may now recall that the previous dentist had suggested crowns but you opted for the fillings. Or you may be told that the dentistry in your mouth is generally poorly done. What do you do now? Local dental societies have peer review committees that will examine your mouth if you feel that you may have been poorly treated. This will cost you little or no money. You may in fact find that the work in your mouth is adequate after all.

You may receive bad news from a specialist. For example a periodontist may suggest that all of the teeth in one jaw need to be extracted and replaced by dental implants. This opinion may surprise you since you expected that only 1 or 2 teeth needed to be extracted. Your first step should be to discuss the options with the general dentist that referred you for the implants or whatever other treatment was required. If you are still confused then ask your dentist to refer you to another specialist. Often times each specialist will have a different opinion. Again it is usually best to take both opinions to your dentist and have him help you decide what is best for you. Ultimately you must be comfortable with the decision. **Remember that dentistry and medicine is an art based on science.** Consequently 2 dentists will suggest 2 different plans but they will only differ in minor respects. Each plan is an appropriate solution to the problem albeit different.

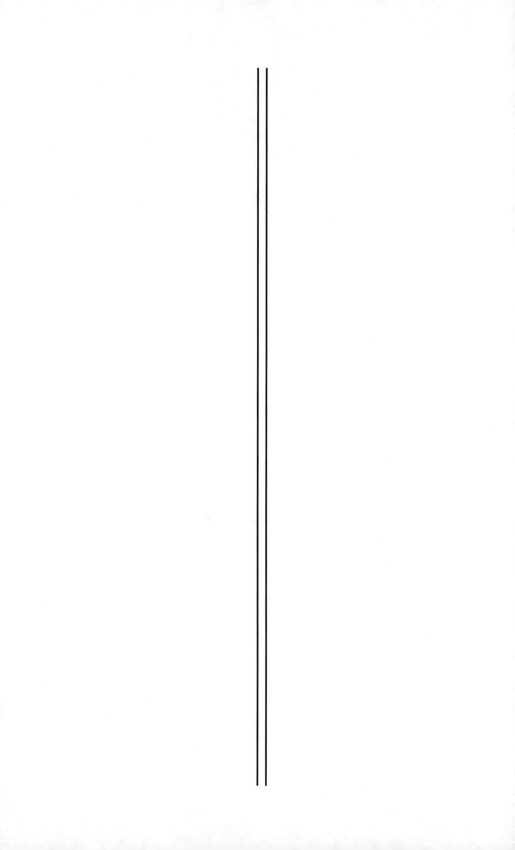

| CHAPTER 7 | What to Expect from Specialists |

The specialties recognized by the American Dental Association are: Periodontics, Endodontics, Orthodontics, Oral and Maxillo Facial Surgery, Pediatric Dentistry, Prosthodontics, Oral Pathology, Public Health and Dental Radiology.

Generally to be considered a dental specialist the dentist advertises his practice being "limited to ..." the particular specialty. This means he limits his practice to this particular area of dental medicine. It also means that this dentist received post graduate training, usually 3 years, in a university setting or a hospital/university setting. It also means that the dentist received a certificate recognizing the successful completion of the required training. This post graduate education occurred after receiving a degree from dental school. **Not all specialists are board certified. What does board certification mean? It means that the dentist passed an examination after the completion of his training showing that he has the skill, knowledge and experience of an expert in this field. The dentist receives the distinction of being called a Diplomate of the board of this particular specialty. Being board certified is different from being board qualified or board eligible.** The later simply means that the dentist may, at some point, take the required examination to become certified but has not yet done so.

In some specialties all specialists are board certified while in others, such as in Periodontics, fewer than 60% of the specialists are certified. Why is this the case? This is true because in some specialties, such as in Periodontics, the exam is complex and time consuming. In Periodontics the candidate first must pass a comprehensive written exam. After successfully doing that the candidate had to submit 3 cases representing the successful treatment of 3 patients with advanced periodontal disease. The case reports included X-rays and photographs before, during and after treatment. The candidate then completed a 2 day oral examination. Recently, the case submission part was eliminated to make the exam less complex and to encourage more periodontists to take the exam since at that point only 30% of the periodontists where board certified.

How do you find a specialist? Usually your general dentist will refer you to a specialist. This is usually a good referral especially if you are happy with your dentist since he will refer you to someone with a similar practice style, personality and fee structure. But not in all cases will this be the best person to treat your problem since your dentist may simply refer you to a specialist he "likes" and is friendly with. You may want to ask your dentist for more than one name and then ask your dentist to tell you about each one and how they might be different and why one of them may be best qualified to help with your problem. If you have dental insurance you may want to know if the specialist is a participant in the plan you have. You may choose to see a specialist who is not in your plan if cost is not a primary consideration. Also consider that treatment provided by the specialist may be a one time experience.

You may also ask about the credentials of each specialist. Meaningful credentials are board certification, experience and appointments at hospitals or dental schools. Appointments are simply an indication that the institution the doctor is appointed to has verified his credentials for appointment and that he has maintained those credentials. Go to the internet and check out the credentials of each specialist. Look for board certification, year of graduation, teaching positions, articles published in the dental literature, and honors received. Most dentists now have web sites and although they are generally self serving they will give you information like location, parking, services available, type of staff, and handicap access. When you call to schedule the appointment ask if they have received your X-rays and other information from your dentist.

Typically you can expect to fill out a comprehensive health history and dental history including your chief complaint. The specialist will then review this material with you and should ask you about any special concerns you might have such as fear of dental injections, fear of surgery, concerns about the impact of treatment on other medical problems you have, etc.

You will then have a clinical exam and required tests, photographs, additional X-rays, models, etc. It may be recommended that a cone beam CT scan be done. This is often done prior to doing dental implants, orthodontics and even in some endodontic practices. Ask if the CBCT is absolutely necessary. In many cases the scan is indispensible but you must also consider the cost. Ask about costs when you make the appointment.

In most cases, especially when the patients' problem is complex, you will be asked to return for a consultation after the specialist has had time to look at the diagnostic materials collected at your exam and has had time to discuss the findings with your dentist. At the consultation the specialist will discuss his findings, give you a diagnosis and outline and explain the options for treatment including the risks, costs, prognosis and best alternatives. You may want to think about all of this or your choice may be clear and you may be motivated to proceed immediately.

Typically the office should be neat, clean and modern in appearance although these things are not as important as your impression of the individual dentist and his staff. You should see evidence that sterile technique and aseptic technique is a rule in the practice. Note if the doctor and his assistants put on new gloves when they enter your treatment room. There is more information about sterility in chapter 5.

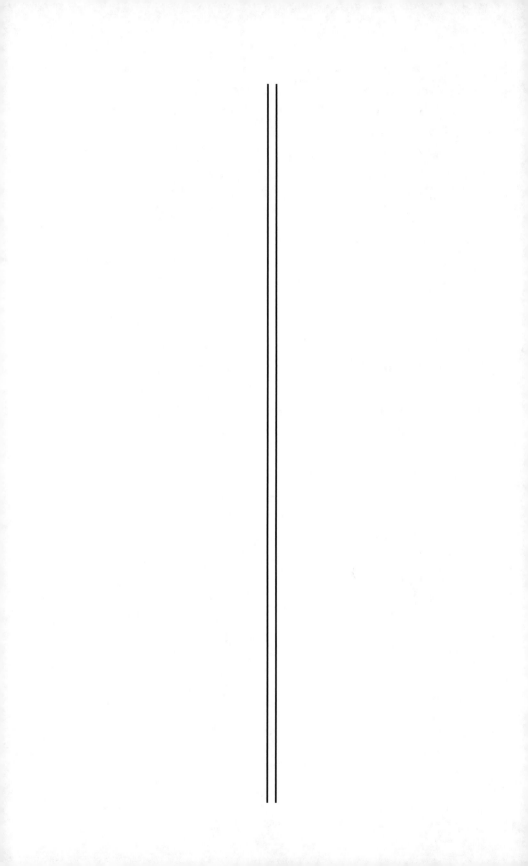

CHAPTER 8   Questions to Ask About the
                Diagnosis and Treatment Plan

Regarding the diagnosis, you can ask how certain the specialist is about the diagnosis and what other diagnoses can be considered. Of course you will typically be told about alternative treatment plans. For example when seeking an opinion about treating periodontal disease you can choose between surgical and non surgical treatment. When seeking an opinion about replacing missing teeth alternative plans will include implant supported restorations or restorations not supported by implants. Bridges are either fixed or removable. Removable bridges may be partial or complete. The complete removable bridge is called a full denture.

You may be told that one or more teeth need to be extracted. Why would a tooth need to be extracted even it is not hurting? In some instances the tooth is broken or decayed extensively and can not be restored to function. In other cases the bone supporting the tooth has been lost due to periodontal disease and the tooth has become very loose making it useless. There are some cases where an X -ray shows infection caused by a dead nerve but the bone loss is so extensive that the result of doing endodontics will be questionable. In other cases the tooth or teeth have so many problems that the dentist believes that extracting the tooth or several teeth is the best option.

In this case you may discuss what resolving the problems entail and you may choose to do so rather than extract the teeth. In summary when many dental problems are present you will usually have several solutions. Make a decision only after getting all relevant information.

Learn about the time, cost and all inconveniences associated with treatment. Ask about risks of non treatment as well as the risks of treatment. In some cases it may seem to be more convenient to do nothing if the damaged teeth aren't troubling you. On the other hand chronically infected teeth can sometimes cause serious health problems. Occasionally the damaged tooth will suddenly start hurting as you begin a trip. The changes in air pressure in airplane cabins during flight may cause an acute flare up at an inopportune time.

If you are diagnosed with a periodontal problem you will be given options regarding surgical or non surgical treatment. Removing a tooth with a poor periodontal prognosis versus doing extensive surgical treatment is a common conundrum. Is it better to remove the tooth and place an implant or make a fixed bridge? In later chapters I will go into greater detail about periodontal and implant treatment in particular. If you wish you may reference these chapters at this time.

When having orthodontic treatment you may choose to have teeth extracted to reduce crowding. Typically the 4 bicuspids will be removed to help with crowding.

You may also have the opportunity to choose between invisible appliances (Invisalign) or traditional appliances (wires and bands also called a fixed appliance). The best choice is what is appropriate for you.

Often there are choices regarding the type of anesthesia to be used. Do you prefer a local anesthetic, intravenous sedation or general anesthesia? Almost all dental procedures are done with local anesthesia. This is the safest and least costly alternative for most patients. However some patients are moderately apprehensive and can be helped with nitrous oxide, a very safe gas, also called laughing gas. Other patients who are very frightened may require I.V. sedation with valium and other sedative drugs. This experience is safe when administered by a specialist trained in anesthesia but not as safe as local anesthesia. This is the same modality you typically experience when having a colonoscopy. You will have no memory of the procedure. General anesthesia is rarely used except for the most complicated procedures such as orthognathic surgery or for medically compromised patients who are best treated in a controlled hospital environment.

Do you require medical consultation? If your medical history is negative you will not need to see your physician. However if the treatment plan is extensive and your health history is not ideal then seek medical clearance. For example insulin dependent diabetics, smokers, patients with chronic cardiac disease, patients with compromised circulation, all have potential problems with healing. Certain medications: anti coagulants, aspirin, plavix, steroids, as well as certain blood pressure medications can dictate modification in dental treatment.

Patients who have had radiation to the upper or lower jaw are at risk of bone necrosis or bone death after dental surgery. Recently we have read that the long term use of bisphosphonates (drugs like Fosamax for osteoporosis) can put patients at risk of osteonecrosis of the jaw after dental surgery. This disease is called ONJ and is more likely to occur when these drugs were administered intravenously for the treatment of cancer that had spread to the bones. However, poor healing of the bone may occur even with oral administration of Fosamax especially if the patient has been taking the drug for more than three years.[7] Other medications such as those used for chemotherapy can complicate dental treatment so the treatment must be coordinated between the dentist and the oncologist.

---

7   Marx R E , et.al. Bisphosphonate induced exposed bone of the jaw J of Oral and Maxillo Facial Surgery 2005;63:1567

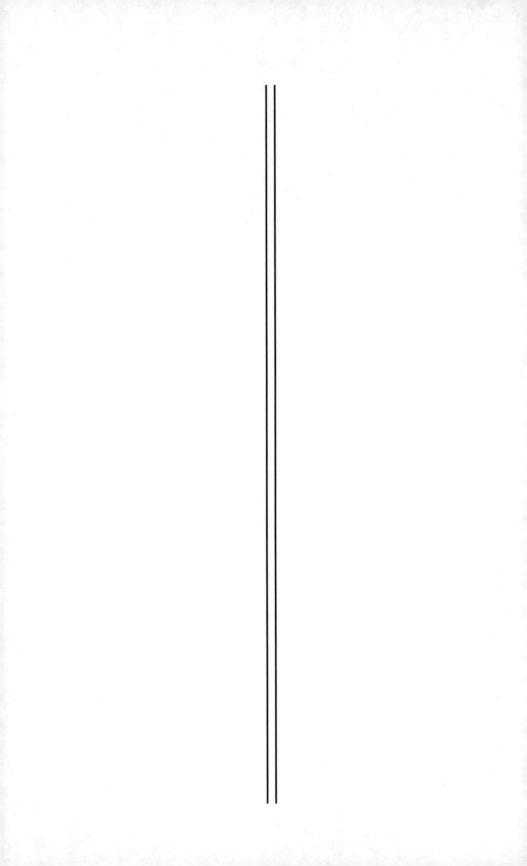

CHAPTER 9

How to Deal With Costs and Payment

Should I buy insurance? Can treatment be financed? The dentist will give you a fee for treatment. This should be given to you in writing and should reflect what each procedure costs.

You may be asked to make a payment arrangement. If this is not done then you should ask how the fee can be paid.

If you have dental insurance the dentist may submit a pre determination of benefits. After a few weeks you and the dental office will receive a written statement reflecting the benefits to be paid by your insurance. This will generally be part of the fee charged by the dentist. The percentage paid varies with the quality of the insurance plan and the fee profile of the dentist. You may ask the dentist if they will accept payment from the insurance so that you will merely pay the balance. If the dentist is a participating dentist in your insurance plan then he will only require you to pay the balance. Can you ask the dentist if he will accept payment from the insurance company as payment in full? This is rarely done since the insurance company considers this "waver of co payment" and it is against the law.

If you do not have insurance then you may ask if you can make installment payments. Some dentists use Care Credit which is a finance company. Care Credit will pay the dentist the full fee up front. You will be given either 6 months or a year to pay back the fee to Care Credit interest free. Of course this is possible because the dentist will be paying the interest. If you fail to make all payments on time you will be subject to a large interest payment to

Care Credit so beware. Some dentists may offer you a discount if you pay the entire fee in advance.

How do you know if the fee is fair? If you have dental insurance and the dentist participates in your plan, he must charge the fee that the insurance company assigns for each procedure.

If you are being treated by a dentist who does not participate in any plans then the dentist can charge whatever fee he or she feels the service merits. Remember that you are not purchasing a product. If you are having teeth capped or an implant placed, you are not paying for the cap or implant but rather for the service that the dentist provides. For example one dentist may spend much more time planning the case, may use a more expensive lab or may be using a more expensive implant. The fees assigned for various services by the insurance companies are low end fees. Dentists that agree to accept these fees are counting on doing a large volume of dental work to compensate for the lower fees. Do you prefer to see a dentist who charges a lower fee if he is much busier and will probably spend less time doing procedures? The dentist may participate in plans with lower fees because he is not busy and hopes to attract more patients. The insurance plans will advertise his name as a participating dentist. Why isn't this dentist busy enough? Is there something wrong with the level of care he provides? I think that most plan dentists provide an adequate level of dental care. I would also expect that dentists not participating in plans and charging higher fees are providing the highest level of care. If you have no choice because your financial resources are limited, these are moot points but you usually get what you pay for. However if the dentist is charging you 2 or 3 times the fee that the insurance company prescribes then you might want to discuss this with his staff.

Sometimes a very good dentist may charge twice what the insurance company dictates. If you are having major dental work done and if the fee is very large, then you may want to get a second opinion. But remember that each dentist is different and will usually have a plan that is somewhat different and the fees will be different as well. Dentistry is an art based on science and again you are not paying for a product. If you are going to buy a BMW 330xi with standard factory accessories then you can compare prices from one dealer to another since the car will be exactly the same. This will not be so when comparing dental services.

When the total cost is unaffordable you may ask the dentist if he can prioritize the services so that you can do some of it now and some next year. In some instances this is possible and in others it is not. For example if you would like to have implants done to replace 2 missing back teeth where one missing tooth is in the upper jaw and the other is in the lower then it is reasonable that you may do each project separately. On the other hand if you would like to have 2 implants done to give your upper denture more support then both implants must be done at the same time. Each treatment plan is unique and no generalization can be made. Of course changing the plan can result in the largest change in the fee. If a patient can not afford a denture supported by implants the patient may choose to tolerate the denture and have the implants done when possible.

If you do not have dental insurance how can you purchase it. The best insurance plans are provided by your employer. This is especially true if you work for a large corporation. There are some companies that allow contributions to a flex spending program for dental care. These plans are best because both the employee and employer pay for it. It is also tax free income. Good dental insurance is very expensive because, unlike medical insurance, patients will use their dental insurance for elective items. You may be able to buy insurance as part of a group such as AARP or alliances in the area you work in (i.e. carpenters association).

You can purchase a reduced fee agreement from dental plans.com. You will find it on the internet. It is inexpensive. The cost is about $109 per person or $139 per family. This is not insurance. It works by enrolling dentists who agree to work for a lesser than average fee. For example most dentists charge $168 dollars for a 3 surface filling; a plan dentist agrees to charge only $90. How can the dentist discount the filling by almost 50%? Because the plan will advertise his name and his practice and he hopes to do a larger volume of dental treatment. There are no claims to file. You pay the dentist the total but reduced fee for service.

The problem is most dentists do not participate in this plan. You can check on the internet to see which dentists in your town participate in dentalplans.

com There are several plan names such as the Northeast Dental Plan and others under the dentalplans.com title. They will advertise names of dentists participating in your area as well as the fees they charge for specific services.

CHAPTER 10

What to Expect When Having Oral Surgery

When oral surgery is done by a general dentist it is usually done with local anesthesia. This is the same technique as used when you are having a filling done except a longer acting and more profound drug may be used. For example when having simple restorative dentistry done the anesthetic may be Carbocaine without adrenalin. This means that the numbness will last 30 to 45 minutes. For longer procedures an anesthetic like Xylocaine with a small amount of adrenalin (one part of adrenalin to 100,000 parts of anesthetic) is often used. The adrenalin allows the numbness to last longer. In the upper jaw it will last for 60 minutes and in the lower it will last for 3 hours. The adrenalin also closes the small blood vessels in the area injected and therefore reduces bleeding allowing the dentist to see better. This is a good thing. Healthy patients can have some adrenalin without any serious side effects. Occasionally some of the anesthetic will be injected into blood vessels accidently. This will cause a temporary increase in blood pressure and heart rate. This can be slightly unpleasant but the effect wears off in about 2 to 3 minutes. Don't panic! However medically compromised patients such as those with heart problems related to heart rate and rhythm or patients with poorly controlled blood pressure are often treated with minimal adrenalin or no adrenalin since an accidental intra vascular injection could exacerbate their medical problem. Consultation between the dentist and the physician is mandatory in these cases.

There are some prescription medications that interact poorly with adrenalin (i.e. epinephrine).

Some examples are psychogenic medications like the tricyclic antidepressants or certain blood pressure medications like Metoprolol. Almost all patients can and should have local anesthesia with adrenalin for oral surgery but some patients require the minimum amount possible.

In any event, it is important that the dentist is aware of medication you are taking so that appropriate precautions can be taken. There is no allergy to local anesthesia with the currently used drugs. The most common local anesthetics currently used are Lidocaine and Mepivacaine which are amide type anesthetics. Many years ago, prior to 1967 or so, Novacaine was in use and this type of drug did cause allergic reactions. This drug was an ester type of anesthetic. If you had a true allergic reaction to Novacaine such as hives or a rash then tell your dentist about this.

Some of the topical anesthetics used currently are esters. Allergy to the topical anesthetic is possible.

If the surgery is done by a periodontist the anesthetic is usually local since very few periodontists are trained to use I.V. anesthesia. The training is extensive and requires a special certificate. If necessary the periodontist and the patient may agree to have a dental anesthesiologist provide the required sedation. Periodontists will often use nitrous oxide analgesia. This gas, also called laughing gas, is an analgesic and does create some euphoria (makes you happy). This is a safe drug which is eliminated from the body within 2 minutes with no after effects. You may drive afterward. Some dentists are also trained in sedation by mouth meaning that they can administer or prescribe an oral sedative like Valium or Xanax to be taken along with the nitrous oxide. Typically you may eat before surgery if you are not having I.V. sedation or general anesthesia. You will be instructed not to take aspirin for 10 days before surgery unless aspirin has been prescribed by your physician. In that case check with your physician to determine if it can be stopped or if the dosage can be modified. We have found that taking 81 mg of aspirin will not cause excessive bleeding. I have also found that patients taking Plavix before surgery have only a small increase in bleeding compared to what is normally seen.

Ibuprofen products like Advil will cause prolonged bleeding after surgery. The effect wears off within 24 hours. In this case you should discontinue the ibuprofen a day or two before surgery.

In most cases surgery, be it an extraction, implant surgery or periodontal surgery, is completely painless. You will feel pressure but not pain. If you are a so called "good" patient the pressure will not trouble you. If you are not a "good" patient then nitrous oxide, oral sedation or I.V. sedation will help you to not be aware of or concerned about pressure. Most procedures take from 20 minutes (simple tooth extraction) to 3 hours (placement of 8 implants with bone grafting). With the longer procedures you will find several opportunities to "take a brake" while the dentist is taking X-rays or mixing materials. Remember that you may ask for a brake at any time and you should if you need to.

I once had an experience while doing full mouth periodontal surgery worth relating. The patient requested I.V. sedation and was treated in the hospital. During the procedure the patient complained a bit and I asked the anesthesiologist if the patient was feeling pain. He responded that she wasn't. I asked how he knew that and he commented that she was complaining even when I was doing nothing! In fact she needed to urinate because of all of the I.V. fluids we were giving her. Two nurses escorted her to the ladies room along with her I.V. bottle.

The next day the patient inquired about how she behaved during the surgery. I commented that she did great except when she had to go to the bathroom. She had no memory of this since the I.V. sedation causes amnesia of all events occurring during the procedure. She thought this was really embarrassing.

After the surgery is completed you will be allowed to rest with some ice. We will offer the patient over the counter pain meds like Advil or Tylenol. The patient is always given written instructions clearly explaining post operative care. I go over this orally with each patient.

Patients are given appropriate pain medications and usually antibiotics. Penicillin is the drug of choice after oral surgery. Amoxicillin is sometimes given to a patient who has had a bone augmentation involving the maxillary sinus. Pain medications will range in strength from Advil or the generic ibuprofen to Vicodin. It is best to take pain medications before the pain starts. For example if I do surgery for a patient at 10 am and I expect the numbness to wear off at 1 p.m I will advise the patient to start the pain medication at 12 30 p.m. If the procedure was short in duration and only involved the soft tissue then ibuprofen is usually adequate. I advise patients to start with ibuprofen but if after 20 minutes some pain persists then take 2 times 500 mg of Tylenol on top of the ibuprofen. If both medications fail to work after another 30 minutes then take the prescribed Vicodin or what ever drug was prescribed. Know the maximum amount of pain medication that can be safely taken during a 24 hour period. Narcotics can and often cause nausea, dizziness, drowsiness or constipation.

Surgical procedures, especially in the lower jaw and especially if grafting materials are used, will be accompanied by swelling. The swelling occurs the next day and is worse upon arising and then diminishes during the day. Swelling will usually peak 48 hours after surgery and will be gone 5 days later but there is some variation. Patients will sometimes have bruising. This will take 5 to 7 days to resolve. Swelling is minimized by: using ice compresses for 20 minutes each hour after surgery, elevating the head with an extra pillow and reducing activity.

Of course if you have taken an anticoagulant like coumadin and have been advised by your physician and your dentist not to stop it or reduce the dosage, then you will be more likely to have post operative bleeding and hematoma (black and blue turning to green after a few days). This is a special situation and you must be given special instructions about what to do about your anti coagulation meds and how to handle post operative bleeding.

You will generally see the surgeon 7 days later for post operative care including removal of sutures (lay people call them stitches) if they are not resorbable. Often non resorbable sutures are preferred since they cause less inflammation. Sutures that dissolve away seem preferable but I use them mostly when placing sutures in areas beneath the skin or gum tissue. Occasionally sutures made from medical grade Gore Tex are used. Nothing sticks to this material so the sutures may remain under the gum tissue for several weeks without causing irritation. These sutures are more costly than silk, nylon or gut sutures. At 7 days post surgery, the area is not fully healed. Patients often ask how long will healing take. That depends on how one defines healing. The surgeon defines completed healing as when the tissues have completely regenerated. The soft tissue or gum tissue is healed in about 3 weeks depending of the size of the area. The hard tissue, bone, takes on average 3 to 6 months to heal. For example when doing an implant in the lower jaw, healing of the bone about the implant is 65% completed in 3 months but healing in the upper jaw will take about 6 months. If you define healing as when can I, the patient, expect to no longer have discomfort then that may be in as little as 24 hours or it may be as long as 2 to 3 weeks. Again it depends on the procedure and the surgeon can usually predict average healing time.

Will you develop infection after surgery? This would be uncommon after dental surgery in a healthy patient because the mouth has very good blood supply to support healing. However if your immune system is compromised by diabetes, smoking or other illnesses then infection is more common. The use of steroids after surgery reduces pain and swelling but will make the patient more susceptible to infection since steroids reduce the effectiveness of the immune system. All things considered, oral surgery has a faster recovery time than most other surgical areas. For the first week or two it can be an inconvenience since the area can't be put at rest. You will need to speak and eat. Certainly you will need to eat softer foods and sometimes only liquids at first. If only a quarter or half of your mouth was treated then you will eat on the other side. You should plan oral surgery, if possible, at a convenient time. I would not have oral surgery done on New Years Eve. Don't have surgery the day before the doctor leaves on vacation. Ask about things like this when planning the surgery. Occasionally I have had patients tell me at the completion of a surgical procedure that they will be away the following week.

Complications are not common. However what are the more frequent complications?

Pain and swelling are normal but extensive swelling and resultant pain is not. If the swelling gets worse on the third day after surgery, call the doctor. This may be related to infection or bleeding under the soft tissues. If it is infection, the surgeon will anesthetize the area and debride or clean it. He may also change the antibiotic and take a culture to see if an unusual bacterium is the cause. If it is a hematoma or blood clot then he will either leave it alone or drain it if it doesn't resolve in 2 weeks.

Occasionally a procedure will fail as a result of infection or swelling. A procedure will also fail if the area is traumatized by eating on it or smoking. **Some procedures will need to be redone. A more serious complication is nerve damage. This can occur with the removal of an impacted lower wisdom tooth. It may also occur while placing a dental implant in the lower back portion of the mouth. So it you have numbness that persists in your lower lip or tongue for more than 24 to 48 hours then call the surgeon or dentist who did the surgery. In most cases the numbness is transitory. If it is slowly getting better the chances are good that it will resolve. If it is not improved after 2 weeks, a specialist in nerve injury should be consulted. In some cases if 3 weeks or more pass without intervention there may be no chance to repair the damage**. I believe that the current use of CT scans will help surgeons to be more aware of potential nerve injury. Typically there are one or two oral surgeons in your area that your dentist can refer you to for this problem. Severe bleeding that persists after applying pressure for a couple of hours is a serious complication. By severe I mean bleeding that persists even while you are holding gauze tightly on the area or bleeding causing your mouth to fill with blood. You will need to see your dentist. He will numb the area, apply hemostatic materials (collagen sponges) and resuture.

In some cases it may be necessary to construct a stent which is an acrylic plate that will cover the area and place constant pressure on it for several days. I had this happen once in my 40 years of practice. The bleeding may be so severe that going to a hospital emergency room is required. This would be a wise thing to do if you can not contact your dentist immediately or if it is late at night and you do not live close to the dentist's office. It is smart to go to a hospital that has an oral surgery teaching program. On Long Island this would be Long Island Jewish Hospital in New Hyde Park or Nassau County Medical Center in East Meadow. The hospital should have a dental residency program where the resident will be on the premises and will be able to help immediately. At the hospital the amount of blood loss can also be determined.

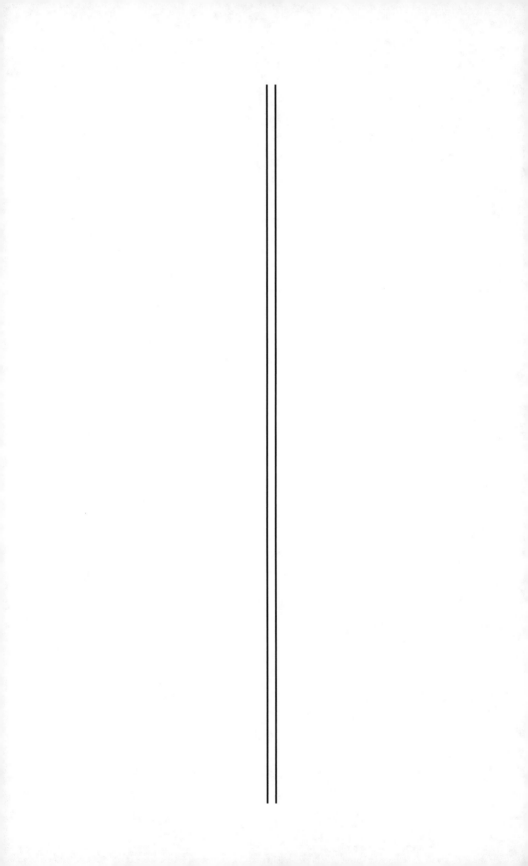

CHAPTER 11

How to Benefit From Periodontal Treatment

What is periodontal treatment all about? Patients are referred to a periodontist for many reasons. You may be referred for the treatment of gum disease. Periodontists also see patients for dental implant placement, for crown lengthening and for cosmetic dental procedures.

Dental implants are discussed elsewhere in this book in chapter 10.

Crown lengthening surgery is a common surgical procedure done in periodontal practices. The general dentist refers the patient for crown lengthening when a tooth is badly broken or decayed so that little of the tooth is exposed above the gum. This makes it difficult for the dentist to make a cap or crown that will bond to the remaining tooth. Caps are held on by friction more than by cement or bonding materials. Crown lengthening surgery involves making the tooth longer to provide more retention for the cap. The periodontist, or dentists if they choose to do this, must first remove an appropriate amount of gum tissue and then flap back the gum to expose the bone so that the required amount of bone can be removed. Typically the dentist requires 4 mm of solid tooth structure exposed above the bone. For example if the tooth is broken such that merely 2 mm of tooth remains above the bone then the dentist must remove 2 additional mm of bone. After the flap is closed with sutures one or more mm of tooth will be exposed above the gum where as before part of the tooth was under the gum. In many cases most of the tooth is fine but one side of the tooth is broken or decayed below the gum and this requires treatment. Crown lengthening is a tedious procedure that requires 30 to 60 minutes and usually costs about as much as a cap.

Are there alternatives? Many dentists use a laser to do crown lengthening. This is acceptable if no bone removal is required. In most cases bone removal is required. If only soft tissue is removed then the soft tissue will grow back to the original position. The final cap will feel uncomfortable because it will interfere with the gum healing. "You can't fool Mother Nature."

There will be no pain during the surgery but expect some swelling and discomfort the next day especially if this in done in a lower molar area.

Periodontists also do cosmetic periodontal surgery. Generally this involves either adding gum tissue or removing gum tissue and sometimes both but for different teeth. For example many patients are referred because recession of the gum and bone (gum recession implies that the bone also receded) made a tooth or several teeth longer and unsightly.

The periodontist is skilled in doing surgical procedures called soft tissue grafts to add back missing gum tissue and to also cover the exposed roots. These procedures are predictable when done by periodontal surgeons who have had experience doing them. **Ask the dentist where he or she was trained to do cosmetic surgery and what his or her success rate has been. Please smile when you ask questions like this.** Some patients present with teeth that are too small or not as long as the same tooth on the other side. This causes a loss of symmetry. This is corrected with crown lengthening as described above.

The treatment of periodontal disease began in antiquity and in 1918 Periodontics became a specialty. The periodontist will initially examine your mouth looking for damage that has been done such as bone loss and gum or gingival recession. The looseness of teeth will be noted. Information will also be collected about causative factors such as amount of plaque and tartar, bite discrepancies, smoking habits and factors in the medical history that may have contributed to the disease. The periodontist will formulate a plan summarizing the treatment required, the prognosis of the teeth (how will they fair in the future) and the fee for treatment.

The initial stage of treatment for adult periodontitis, the most common type of periodontal disease, includes scaling or deep cleaning. This is often done in four visits. One quadrant of teeth is treated at each visit using a local anesthetic. Scaling is used to remove deposits like plaque and calculus from the roots of the teeth. This is difficult to do where the periodontal pockets are deeper than 5 mm especially in the back of the mouth. This may be done by the periodontist or by the hygienist. Many hygienists are certified to use local anesthesia and/or nitrous oxide analgesia. The scaling is done with an ultra sonic instrument with water spray and /or with hand instruments called scalers or curettes. During these initial visits, oral hygiene instruction is also done. As cited earlier the patients' interest and ability to remove the bacterial plaque that reforms every 24 hours determines whether inflamation of the gums and bone will recur. To a large extent you are in control of your own destiny. Failure to perform daily plaque control as instructed will result in failure of periodontal treatment.

After the first stage of treatment is completed the periodontist will evaluate the results to determine if bleeding on probing has been eliminated or at least reduce. If not then additional scaling or pre surgical treatment may be rendered. The periodontist will also recommend a final surgical plan. He may decide that fewer teeth require surgery. Usually the surgical plan remains the same but the soft tissues are healthier and can be more effectively treated with surgery since there will be little bleeding from healthy gum tissue. The goal of periodontal surgery for deep periodontal pockets is to reduced the depth of the pockets, regenerate lost bone if possible and render the tissues (bone and gum tissue) healthier. How is this done? After giving local anesthesia an incision is made and the gum is reflected back to expose the roots of the teeth and the surrounding bone. With good access and visibility the roots can be meticulously cleaned of any remaining deposits. At this time the bone is evaluated and typically the periodontist will find small craters or holes in the bone around the teeth. If the craters are small, less than 3 mm deep, they are filed down to eliminate spaces where bacteria and unhealthy tissue can grow.

If the craters are deep, 3 mm or deeper, they will require grafting. Graft materials are available from tissue banks. These bone graft materials are sterile and do not stimulate a rejection phenomena by the patient. The gum tissue is carefully closed over the graft by the surgeon. The patient will not feel the presence of the graft material. It is suggested that the patient not chew on the specific area treated with a bone graft for 8 weeks. Bone grafts are successful but success is defined by regenerating 60% or more of the lost bone. Usually bone regeneration will occur but the extent of the regeneration depends on many factors including how well the patient heals. Again results in smokers are less successful. Chewing on the healing area during the first 8 weeks after surgery will cause failure of the graft.

Regeneration procedures have been done by periodontists since the late 1960's. The procedures have become more successful and more sophisticated. Cost depends on how many areas in one quadrant require grafting and what types of materials need to be used. Cost in my office is $950 for the basic procedure and an additional $400 to $500 for materials. These procedures heal with few complications. Swelling for 1 to 3 days may occur but without pain. The most common complication is failure of the graft.

CHAPTER 12

Dental Implants, are they for You?

Are dental implants in your future? Dental implants have become the first option for replacing missing teeth. In the last 25 years millions of implants have been done in this country and around the world. The success rate of dental implants is 90 to 95%. What is meant by success is that after 5 years or longer the implant is firm, without pain or infection and less that 2 mm of bone loss is seen on X-ray.

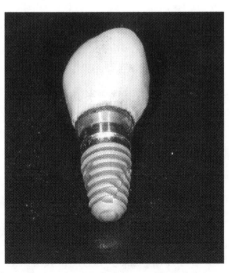

Fig. 3 Photo shows a cap (top 1/3) cemented on an abutment post (middle 1/3 polished titanium). The abutment is screwed into the implant (bottom 1/3, grey threaded screw).

What is a dental implant? (Fig.3). the implant is a screw made of a titanium alloy. The human body does not reject titanium. The surface of the implant receives special treatment to aid in the attraction of bone forming cells. Implants are manufactured in a sterile environment and are delivered to the dentist in a sterile container. The body of the implant can vary in size from 7 to 18 mm in length and from 1.8 mm to 6 mm in diameter. The most commonly placed implants are 4 mm in diameter and 13 mm in length.

The implant is usually placed by a periodontist or an oral surgeon. However some general dentists also place implants. Generally the placement protocol involves a surgical procedure where the gum tissue is reflected back to expose the bone. The surgeon typically has planned the procedure using X-rays and some times a CT scan to measure the amount of bone available. A new socket is carefully prepared to fit the planned implant. The implant is carefully placed into the socket so that the top of the implant is flush with the crest of bone. Placement of the implant is accomplished with a special dental motor which carefully controls the speed and force of insertion. Preparation of the socket as well as insertion of the implant must be done precisely according to a time tested protocol to insure proper healing of the bone such that the bone adheres to the implant. Cold sterile water is used to prevent over heating of the bone while the site is prepared for the implant. Special implant drills are used to insure exact sizing of the implant site. **This protocol is different from that used in the early years of implant surgery, 1950 to 1970, when high speed drills were used. The use of high speed drills, 200,000 revolutions per minute, inadvertently caused the bone to die back from the implant during the healing process. This die back was caused by excessive heat generated during the preparation. Because of the die back the implant healed with a soft tissue capsule around it rather than the direct bone to implant contact that is attained with the modern protocol. Implants done with this high speed protocol failed after five years or earlier because of the lack of direct bone to implant contact where as the modern implant potentially will remain healthy and functional indefinitely.**

A healing period of 3 to 6 months is then required for the bone and implant to integrate. The surgeon evaluates the success of the implant in several ways. First an X-ray is taken. The X-ray should show bone to implant contact with no dark space between the bone and implant. Sometimes an implant will look well integrated on X-ray but not be integrated. The surgeon will manually test to see that there is no movement. Tapping firmly on the implant should not cause any discomfort.

If the implant or implants pass these tests then the restorative or general dentist continues treatment. This treatment involves fabrication of a post which is screwed into the implant. This post is usually custom made. Then a cap or crown is made to fit on the post. The crown is either cement retained or screw retained at the discretion of the dentist. As you can see the surgeon inserts an implant which does not include a post and crown. It would be impossible to insert the 3 components in one piece. There are several reasons this is not possible the most significant of which is that the tooth space required is different for each case and so the post and cap must be custom made for each patient.

An implant may be used to replace one missing tooth or many missing teeth. In some cases the patient has lost all of their natural teeth and may be a candidate for 6 to 10 implants placed to support 10 to 12 caps. In other situations it may be suitable for a patient to have a denture made and 2 to 4 implants used to support the denture. How one determines what is appropriate is beyond the scope of this book. Suffice it to say that it depends on how much bone and gum tissue is missing. It also depends on the requirements of the individual patient. By requirements I mean esthetics, function and finances.

The surgery is usually done with local anesthesia and is painless. The surgical visit may take from 45 minutes to 3 hours depending on how many implants are being placed, how many teeth are being extracted and if grafting is required to increase the volume of hard and soft tissue. If there is no medical contra indication to having a tooth extracted then there should be no contra indication to having a dental implant placed. How does one decide between an implant and a bridge? It is usually best to trust the opinion of your dentist. Generally if ample bone is present and if the adjacent teeth are in good repair then an implant is a good choice.

What do implants cost? Again it depends on many factors like who is doing the treatment as well as where it is being done. Generally the surgical placement of an implant will cost $1500 to $2000. The restorative phase will cost about $2400 per implant. Usually dental insurance will pay a small part of this. Medical insurance rarely pays for this service. If you have little money to spend on this type of dentistry consider having it done in a dental clinic at your local dental school. This will not be at all convenient but it will be less than half the cost. Financing is available in many dental offices. Care Credit is a popular credit company. Typically the company pays the dentist up front and the patient gets 6 months to a year to pay off the debt. You may have seen advertising for implants being done for $395. The restoration must be done at this facility. The total cost is advertised as $1695. How can they do it at this price? Firstly they do a large volume. Also keep in mind that you are not buying an implant. You are having a service performed. Often times the surgeon who does the implant and the dentist who restores the implant are employees in this type of volume practice. If you have problems with the implant or the restoration later on the dentists who did the work may be long gone. In my practice, and this is common in quality private practices, I will do the implant over at no charge if the implant fails. This means that I will charge the patient for the actual cost of the implant which ranges from $300 to $400.

Millions of implants are being done annually because they are the most acceptable way to replace missing teeth. The procedure is costly but the benefits out way the cost. Pick a dentist to carefully and thoroughly diagnose and plan your implant experience. Find a dentist with good credentials and training in implant dentistry. Occasionally you will find a dentist who has had excellent training in both the surgical placement of the implant and the restoration of the teeth.

This is convenient but there are few dentists expert in both phases of implant dentistry.

More typically you will try to find an implant surgeon and restorative dentist who have done many successful cases together.

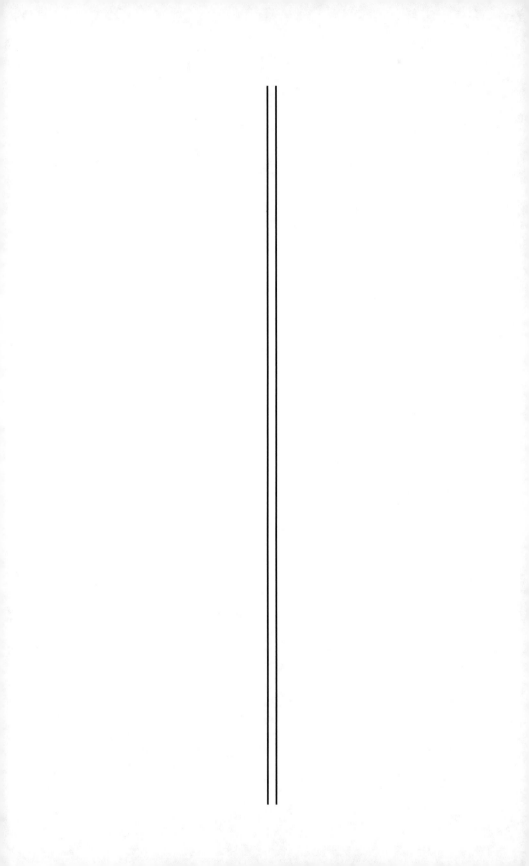

CHAPTER 13

Endodontics or Root Canal Tratment

This is a popular specialty in our society. How many jokes have we heard beginning with "I'd be happy to have a root canal" rather than... The pulp chamber of the tooth is the most internal layer which contains the blood vessels and nerves which give the tooth the capacity to feel pain. Decay progressing to the pulp will cause a tooth ache. In time the pulp will die or become necrotic. The death of the pulp will eventually result in infection of the pulp. This may or may not cause a toothache but it will cause a loss of bone at the apex of the tooth. In some cases the infection will travel to the soft tissue surrounding the apex. In an upper tooth this will result in swelling of the face sometimes including the upper eye. In rare cases the infection can travel to the brain. In the lower jaw infection may result in swelling of the cheek and in rare cases swelling of the floor of the mouth causing difficulty in breathing. Antibiotics and draining of the abscess will help but will not cure the problem.

The cures for the problem are removal of the tooth or removal of the dead pulp. Removal of the pulp is what the endodontist or root canal specialist does.

What is a root canal? Anatomically the root canal is the canal which leads from the pulp, which is in the center of the crown of the tooth, to the apex or tip of the root.

Once the dentist or endodontist (if you chose to see a specialist) opens into the pulp drainage will occur and relief of pain is immediate in most cases.

Endodontic or root canal treatment involves removal of all of the dead soft tissue in the pulp and root canal or canals. Other events can cause death of the nerve. The most common cause other than decay is a fractured tooth.

Many teeth, in particular the molars, have several root canals. Many of these canals are small and curved making removal of the dead tissue challenging. Modern Endodontists generally use a microscope to aid in seeing small canals and enable proper treatment of the tooth.

Many dentists do root canal treatment for their patients but often refer out molar root canals because of the technical difficulty involved. Treatment is not painful. Root canal treatment is often done in one visit. Of course a tooth with one canal, like a front tooth, will take less time to treat than a molar. Cost is generally $1300 for a molar done by an endodontist. A front tooth may cost $1000. Specialists who participate in an insurance plan will charge less for a molar root canal possibly $900.

In many cases the general dentist will suggest removal of the tooth and placement of a dental implant. Which is the better alternative? If the tooth is badly broken or badly decayed then restoring it may be questionable. An implant will be a better choice if there is adequate bone to place an implant.

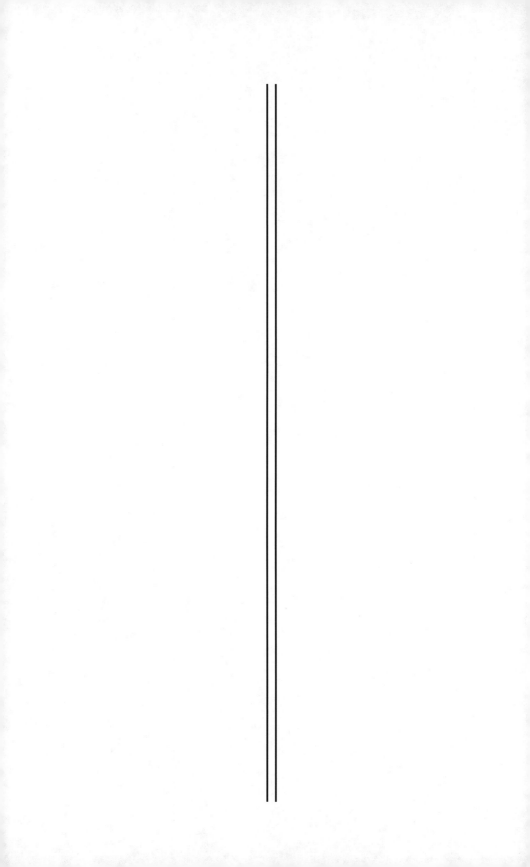

CHAPTER 14   Maintenance Care,
                             is it Important?

Regular maintenance care is the most important behavior needed to arrest periodontal disease. It is also helpful in preventing other dental diseases such as decay and oral cancer. The cost of maintenance care, probably $500 a year for 4 visits, will save you many thousands of dollars over a lifetime compared to showing up only when it hurts. Regular professional maintenance care can be the most effective aid in saving your teeth.

What exactly should be done at a maintenance or recall visit? Of course your teeth will be cleaned. All root surfaces will be scaled with special attention given to areas where the pocket is deeper than the normal 1 to 3 mm. Finally the teeth will be polished. However it is more than just a "cleaning". The dentist or hygienist will re examine the teeth and gums for recurrent disease or new disease. It is common for deep pockets (5 to 10 mm) to have recurrent pocketing years after surgical treatment. Finding this early and treating it with aggressive scaling and local drug delivery can negate the need for more surgery. Some times X-rays will be taken. Certainly oral hygiene instruction will be reviewed if there are signs that the patient has been lax. An oral cancer screening exam should be done at each recall visit. This will include careful inspection of the tongue, floor of the mouth, gingiva and oral mucosa for suspicious lesions such as non healing ulcers. An ulcer that has been present for more than 2 weeks should be evaluated. Patients at higher risk are smokers, drinkers and black males.

Suspicious lesions should be biopsied or referred to an oral surgeon for biopsy.

Studies have shown that having 3 month recare visits is appropriate for periodontal patients. A study done in Sweden involving 600 patients showed that the 3 month recall completely arrested periodontal disease. On the other hand the control group of patients who had recalls once a year regressed to the pre periodontal treatment status. This is to say that all of the progress made by having periodontal surgery was lost during a 6 year period for those patients who presented only annually for recall. They noted that the 3 month recall group also had fewer cavities.[8]

Who should be doing the recall treatment? In most periodontal offices as well as in most general practices the dental hygienist does the scaling. The dentist will do an exam after the hygienist is finished. The dentist or the periodontist if that is the case will not necessarily examine the patient on each recall visit. Of course if the hygienist detects a problem then the dentist or periodontist will certainly examine the patient. It will also depend on the patient. If we are seeing a patient who has had severe and refractory dental disease then it would be appropriate for the dentist to see the patient for evaluation on each visit. Legally in many states, the dentist doesn't have to be in the office physically while the hygienist is doing scaling or cleaning. In New York State the dentist must be available (just a few minutes away) in case the patient needs to see the dentist. The hygienist is a licensed professional. The state board of education determines what the hygienist may do under general supervision versus direct supervision. For example the hygienist may be licensed to administer local anesthesia but may only do so if the dentist is physically in the office. **Should the periodontal patient see the general dentist or the periodontist for recalls? Usually it is appropriate for the patient to alternate 3 month recalls. In this way the periodontal staff looks after the periodontal condition and the general dental staff checks for cavities and takes X-rays.**

---

8   Axelsson P & Lindhe J Effects of Controlled Oral Hygiene. Results after 6 Years. J Clin Perio 1981;8:239

CHAPTER 15	Have You Been Mistreated? Should You Sue Your Dentist?

There are several options depending on how you believe you were mistreated. If the problem is relatively minor, such as you are unhappy with the color of a crown or you are unhappy with the sensitivity you have had after periodontal surgery, you may want to mention it to the dentist. The dentist may say that there is nothing that can be done to improve the condition or the dentist may say that under the circumstances this is the best he was able to do. You might feel that the dentist has usually met or exceeded your expectations in the past. You might simply tell the dentist that you are not happy with the result but you appreciate the work he has done in the past and will live with this result.

On the other hand, the results of treatment may be unacceptable. For example the new bridge was very extensive and expensive and you are totally uncomfortable with it. The dentist says he can't do it over. You may want to get another opinion. If you are planning on possibly continuing with this dentist in the future then behave in a pleasant manner. Simply ask the dentist if he will help you get another opinion by giving you a copy of the pertinent records. He must do this in any event. If you see another dentist and are told that the service you received is not acceptable, then you may consider having the dental treatment redone.

What do you do if the cost is considerable? You may call the original dentist and explain the facts about the second opinion. You could also bring in a report from the consulting dentist. The first dentist may now agree to redo the dentistry at no cost. If this is acceptable to you then choose this option. On the other hand the first dentist may not agree with the opinion of the second dentist.

Peer review is the next option to consider when attempting to resolve a dispute with your dentist. All dental societies have a peer review committee in place. The rules are that you must agree in writing to accept the judgment of this committee. You will agree not to pursue a malpractice action in court. The dentist, if he is a member of the dental society and most dentists are, will also accept the determination of the committee. The committee will obtain the records of the dentist. They will then ask you to appear and describe your complaint. The dentists on the committee will examine your mouth. They will also interview the treating dentist. After a while they will render their findings. If they find that the dental treatment was below the standard of care, they will then have the dentist refund all money you paid for this service. That is all you may receive. In other words you can not collect money for the new dentistry but simply what you paid for the original work.

If they find that the dentistry done was acceptable then the matter is over and you will receive no money back.

The final option you may consider is a malpractice action. This is appropriate if you feel that not only is the dental treatment unacceptable but you have suffered an injury that is permanent.

The most common lawsuits in dentistry involve damages like: TMJ pain after having extensive bridge work done, loss of several teeth resulting from failure to diagnose periodontal disease in a timely manner, nerve damage after dental surgery. **If this is the case you will need an experienced dental malpractice attorney. You may find one on the internet but I suggest calling the local bar association for a recommendation.**

In order to prove malpractice four elements must be proven. The elements are duty, breach, injury and proximate cause of the injury. Each of the four elements must be proven. The doctor must have had a duty to provide treatment meeting the standard of care. A departure from the standard of care or a breach must be proven. Damages or injury must have occurred as a result of the departure from the standard of care and the defendant doctor's actions or lack thereof must be the direct cause of the damages. For example it would be a departure from the standard of care if during implant surgery the dentist carelessly allowed a drill to fall into your mouth. However if the drill caused no damages then there would be no grounds for malpractice. It must also be established that the doctor was the direct cause of any damages you sustain. For example, I once served as an expert witness in a malpractice action where a general dentist was sued because a patient developed severe bleeding after surgery done by a periodontist. The patient was not aware of a clotting factor deficiency so the periodontist was not aware of it either. The patient required a blood transfusion and later developed Hepatitis C. She couldn't sue the hospital because the statute of limitations, (one year for a municipal hospital,) had run out. The plaintiff and her attorney sued the general dentist for not making a timely referral thus requiring the plaintiff to require periodontal surgery. The case was not proven since she was referred in a timely manner in my opinion and because the general dentist was not the direct cause of her damages. The hospital was negligent and the tainted blood was the direct cause of her damages. In another case a patient had implant surgery done under general anesthesia. During the procedure the surgeon caused damage to the inferior alveolar nerve resulting in permanent loss of sensation to the patient's lower lip. The patient sued the surgeon and the anesthesiologist. The patient had no reasonable expectation that the anesthesiologist was to protect her or was responsible for the surgery in any way (no duty and no breach of the standard of care). Informed consent is also an issue in professional liability. As an expert witness for 30 years I have seen cases where the patient was properly informed of inherent risks of damages resulting from a procedure. For example impacted lower wisdom teeth are occasionally in intimate contact with the lingual nerve. The patient is informed that the nerve could be permanently damaged as a result of removing the infected wisdom tooth. Injury resulting from removal of this tooth, given that the surgeon met the standard of care in doing the procedure, should not result in a successful malpractice action.

The malpractice attorney will interview you and have you obtain a copy of your dental records. The attorney will have a dental expert review the records and render an opinion as to whether malpractice is evident. If the expert affirms that damages resulted from a deviation from the standard of care resulting in injury to you then the attorney will go forward with the law suit.

The dentist will receive a summons and complaint. His attorney responds and eventually both the dentist and you the plaintiff will appear for an EBT or examination before trial. This usually occurs in the lawyer's office or in the court house. The time involved varies with the complexity of the case but averages 2 hours. After this point the attorney for the defendant dentist and his insurance company decide if they believe that malpractice occurred. In many counties the dentist is interviewed by a malpractice claims committee which is part of the local dental society. This committee renders an opinion as to whether the case should be defended (they believe that the dentist acted properly under the circumstances) or settled. If the case is settled the attorney receives one third of the award. If the case is going to trial then a trial date is set. This process from the time the summons is served to the trial date may take 3 or 4 years. At trial each side will present witnesses including you the plaintiff and the dentist. The trial itself will take 1 or 2 days.

You can see that going ahead with a malpractice suit takes a great deal of time and effort. If you have been advised by qualified dental experts and attorneys that your injury is significant and a direct result of the actions of your dentist, then proceed. However suing for dental malpractice for lesser issues (you're unhappy with the dental work but you have suffered no injury) is inappropriate in my opinion. Another fact worthy of mention is that in most jurisdictions juries usually find in favor of the defendant dentist or physician as the case may be .Small claims court is an option but the maximum award would be $3000. The dentist will be represented by an attorney. It is unlikely that you can get an attorney to represent you there since the award will be relatively small.

CHAPTER 16

What to do if Your Dentist Retires

This situation is treated in the same way as described in chapter 2 "finding a dentist".

If you discover that your dentist is retiring, ask him immediately who he would recommend. Do this even if he has not publicly announced his retirement. Of course once the dentist sells his practice he will be obligated to suggest the dentist who purchased the practice. This person may or may not be the best new dentist for you. Also have your dentist do a complete evaluation of your mouth. Ask what treatment you might expect to have done in the future. Ask the dentist to give you a written treatment plan including costs. You may find this treatment plan useful in the future when a new dentist suggests treatment. Of course it is usually convenient to stay in the practice since you know the staff. Sometimes your dentist will remain in the practice as an employee. If you decide to go elsewhere of course the original practice is obligated to send all records to the new dentist. Leave the door open. Explain that you are simply going for another opinion. The dentist is required to give you a copy of the original X-rays. The law is that the original X-rays are the property of the dentist.

What is the usual course of action if the dentist retires while you are in the middle of having treatment? The law is that if the dentist is retiring voluntarily rather than because of death or illness, then the dentist is obligated to complete any invasive treatment. For example if the dentist has prepared teeth for crowns and placed temporary crowns then the dentist is obligated to complete the treatment. At your discretion you may choose to allow the new dentist to complete the crowns. The same law would apply if orthodontic treatment were in progress.

The orthodontist who started the treatment is obligated to complete treatment. If you were in the middle of having many crowns done and only some were completed but the other teeth were not touched then the retiring dentist is not obligated to finish what had been planned. If the dentist dies and you are left with temporary crowns then you would be entitled to a refund of any money paid. In some cases the practice of the deceased dentist will be acquired by a new dentist. You may choose to have the new dentist complete the treatment. When you continue with a new dentist in a new practice you generally will not receive credit for the treatment previously done.

In rare cases a dentist will have begun extensive treatment, received a significant retainer, and then disappeared from the practice. In this unusual situation you will need an attorney to help you recover some of the funds paid for dental treatment not completed. This unusual scenario is more likely to happen when you have chosen a dentist who is not grounded in the community.

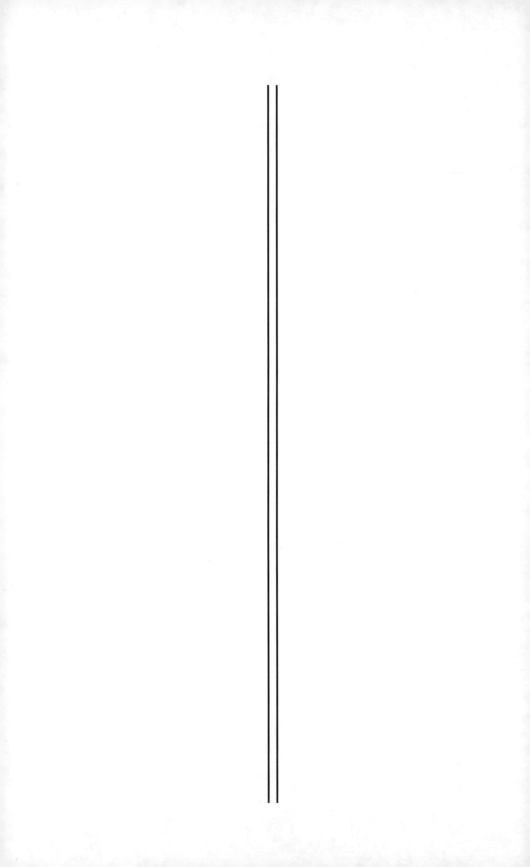

| CHAPTER 17 | Dental Disease Can Affect Your General Health |

Over the past several years a great deal of medical and dental literature has been published associating oral infection and oral inflammation with various health problems.[9] It has been known for years that dental disease associated with significant chronic infection can cause problems with diabetic control. Diabetes can also contribute to periodontal disease being out of control. **More recently studies have shown a high association between chronic dental disease (periodontal disease) and heart attack and stroke. It has been said by some medical experts that inflammation is a greater risk factor for heart attack than high cholesterol.** CPK is a test that measures inflammation. A high CPK has been associated with many diseases. However since inflammatory diseases such as arthritis elevate CPK then it is not specifically predictive for heart attack or stroke. Dental disease has also been associated with low birth weight babies and respiratory disease.

Teeth in poor repair or full dentures make for less effective chewing efficiency which results in choosing a diet that is softer and usually high in refined carbohydrates and sugar. This will contribute to an increase in body fat. We have learned that body fat, especially in the abdomen, is not just added weight (that's bad enough) but it is actually an organ that excretes dangerous chemicals that contribute to inflammation and higher health risks of all kinds. **I believe that having a denture stabilized by 2 implants can be a life saving procedure. It has been shown that an implant supported denture**

---

9   Systemic Conditions Affected by Periodontal Diseases. J. Periodontol. 2000, 71, 880

functions 5 times more efficiently than a denture that is stabilized by denture adhesive. Talking about dental problems that are bad for your health, let's talk about denture adhesives. Denture adhesives contain zinc a chemical that is toxic when ingested.[10] Many denture patients need to wear adhesives. These products melt when the patient drinks hot beverages. Of course the adhesive then runs down into the stomach. The manufacturers claim that if used in the recommended quantity the product is safe. Sadly for many patients the denture just won't stay up so they add more and more product. The temporary solution is to see your dentist as required for relining or remaking the denture. The best solution is to have implants done if possible. Again, 6 to 8 implants will make the denture feel more like having real teeth again. If money and or bone are limited consider just 2 implants to make a big difference.

---

10   Denture Adhesives and Zinc Toxicity. See GlaxoSmithKlein at www.gsk.com

CHAPTER 18 | What Health Issues Can Affect Your Dental Health?

How well diabetes is controlled is measured by the glycolated hemoglobin value which is a measurement of how well controlled the disease is and has been over a period of time.

If your diabetes is out of control you should have only preventive and emergency care until it is under control. Specifically have non surgical periodontal treatment like scaling and home care instruction done frequently. Practice excellent oral hygiene. Postpone elective dental surgery, that is implants and periodontal surgery. Once you are told that the disease is controlled then you may have dental surgery and implants and you will have a normal response to treatment.

Other health problems that will affect dental health are diseases that reduce the potency of the immune system. Examples are HIV, leukemia, nutritional problems and diseases requiring steroid therapy like Chrohn's disease. Chemotherapy also reduces the effectiveness of the immune system. Painful oral ulcerations can occur with chemotherapy making normal oral hygiene difficult. The use of a prescription mouth rinse like Peridex can help with the discomfort as well as helping to control gum disease. Organ transplant patients usually take a drug called Cyclosporine to prevent the organ rejection phenomena. This drug causes severe gum enlargement which will interfere with hygiene. Dilantin, which is used for seizure disorders, also causes gingival enlargement. **Pregnancy, not a disease of course, predisposes women to gingivitis.** This will only happen to women who had some degree of gingivitis before becoming pregnant. Increased hormone levels during pregnancy increases the number of harmful bacteria in the mouth. Pregnancy gingivitis can be avoided by achieving good periodontal health before becoming pregnant and then maintaining good dental hygiene during the pregnancy. Continue to have regular dental cleanings during the pregnancy. Learn to floss your teeth daily even if you didn't previously. The dentist will take precautions like not placing you too far back in the dental chair in the last trimester since this may cause syncope or fainting. Other elective treatment might need to be postponed. This does not relate to the treatment per se but to the drugs that may need to be administered like pain meds or anesthesia. On the other hand it is not safe to have a dental infection. Have your obstetrician and dentist consult about which drugs and procedures are safe and which are not. It is well known that consuming the antibiotic tetracycline will stain the developing teeth of the embryo. Staining only occurs to developing teeth not teeth that are already in the mouth of a child or adult.

The causes of bad breath are multifactorial. Often it is related to dental disease and poor oral hygiene. It may be related to consumption of foods like garlic and onions or smoking. Systemic conditions such as poorly controlled diabetes, lung disease or infected tonsils may also cause bad breath. If the problem persists after eliminating the local factors, then see you physician.

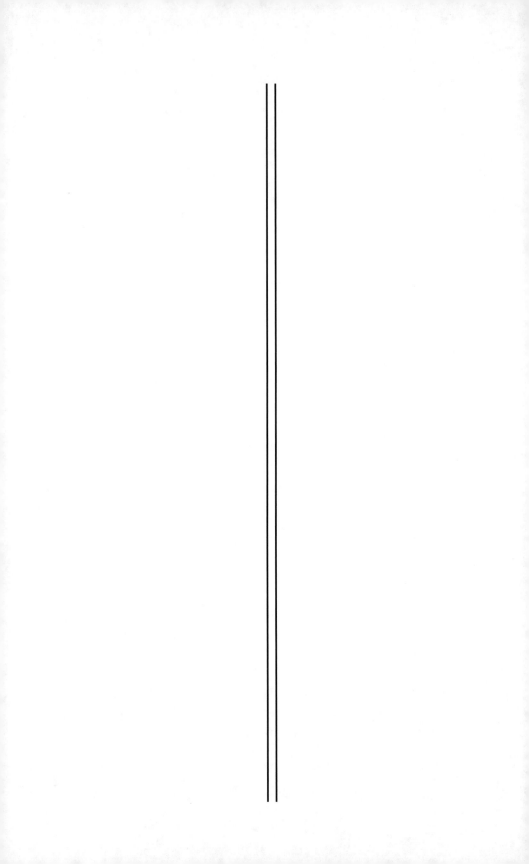

CHAPTER 19 | The Importance of
Your Drug History

The best advice is to tell the dentist about all medications you are taking. After all, this information is confidential. You may be taking a drug, prescribed or otherwise and not know that it could interact with some drug that the dentist is using. The most common example of a drug not revealed in a medical history is aspirin or aspirin products. A person taking 325 mg of aspirin daily to prevent a heart attack is likely to have significant bleeding after dental surgery. The dentist, if aware of the aspirin use, will be prepared to deal with the bleeding. This can be done in many ways. Occasionally the physician will suggest stopping the aspirin 10 days before the surgery. This is done prior to a colonoscopy. It is more difficult to stop bleeding in the colon than in the mouth.

The current thinking is not to stop the aspirin before most dental procedures since this may cause a rebound resulting in an intravascular clot with serious medical consequences.

Instead the dentist may modify the procedure. For example if a patient needs to have all of their teeth extracted, the dentist will do this in 4 visits instead of one visit making it easier to control bleeding. The dentist will typically suture the wound and use hemostatic agents.

Plavix is another drug commonly prescribed for patients who have had stents placed in the coronary arteries. Plavix acts like aspirin. I have found that bleeding during extractions and dental implant surgery is very moderate for patients on Plavix. I have been successful doing surgery for these patients as long as they are not also on aspirin. If they are on both drugs then I will ask the treating physician if it is safe to stop the aspirin and continue the Plavix. Drugs like aspirin or Plavix must be stopped for 10 days to totally eliminate the effect of the drug.

Drugs like Advil or the generic ibuprofen also prolong bleeding after an injury or surgery. However the effects of ibuprofen or similar drugs, also called NSAIDS (non steroidal anti inflammatory drugs) are short acting and are usually gone after 24 hours. Similar drugs are Motrin and Aleve. A similar drug in this regard is Coumadin. While aspirin interferes with bleeding, Coumadin interferes with clotting. Clotting and bleeding are separate mechanisms. These drugs are often called blood thinners by the lay public. They do not make the blood thinner. Anticoagulant drugs simply interfere with the clotting process. If you are taking an anticoagulant your physician will prescribe a blood test monthly which measures the extent of anticoagulation. The therapeutic range for most patients is between 2.5 and 3.5. A higher number means a greater tendency not to clot. This test is called an INR. This is an internationally recognized test that expresses a ratio between the patients' clotting time to a normal clotting time. Another test used is called a prothrombin time test. **You should have your INR done a day or two before seeing your dentist. If the INR is less than 3.5 it will be safe to have your teeth cleaned.** Routine restorative dental procedures like dental injections, fillings and caps cause little or no bleeding so the INR is less relevant. On the other hand dental extractions or having a periodontal surgical procedure becomes a risk for the patient on anti coagulants. An INR of 3.0 may be safe depending on the size of the surgical area. For example having one single rooted tooth extracted will not usually require changing your medication if your INR is 3.0 **On the other hand having multiple extractions often will require a change downward in the INR and this must be done by consultation with your cardiologist.**

There are other medications that may affect your mouth. Blood pressure medications called calcium channel blockers may cause an enlargement of the gum tissue especially if gingivitis is present. This occurs in 40% of the patients taking these drugs. Procardia and Norvasc are 2 examples of this type of medication. Dilantin, a drug used for seizures, also causes significant gum enlargement. **Cyclosporine is a drug used for immuno suppression.**

Patients who have had organs transplanted such as a kidney or liver usually take this drug which also causes enlargement of the gum tissue. Excellent oral hygiene and excellent periodontal health will minimize the enlargement. This is important since the enlarged gingiva will retain more plaque and the generalized inflamation resulting from the plaque retention may endanger the transplanted organ or contribute to other diseases. Patients taking birth control pills need to inform their dentist since taking an antibiotic will reduce the effectiveness of the birth control pill. Dentists often prescribe antibiotics.

Since many medications can affect your dental health it is wise to inform the dentist of any drugs you are taking whether they are prescribed or over the counter. If you take drugs like cocaine or non prescription steroids tell your dentist. Drugs the dentist may prescribe or procedures the dentist may do may be unsafe for you. Remember the information is confidential.

CHAPTER 20

Dental Professionals and Their Training

Why should you, the patient, care about the training of dental professionals? Knowing their training will help you know what to expect from each dental professional and how to interact with them. Careers in dentistry include: dentist with a DDS or DMD degree (there is no difference), dental hygienist with an RDH degree, certified dental assistant with a CDA degree, dental technician with a C.D.T. degree. Dentists and dental hygienists require licenses and a proscribed education program by the State Board of Education. Training as a dental assistant or a dental technician may be received on the job. No license is required for these jobs. However there are formal programs for dental assisting and dental technology. Completion of these programs makes a candidate eligible for certification. Being certified allows the individual to perform duties that an uncertified individual may not perform.

`I will briefly discuss each of these careers. Dentists are college educated first and then go to dental school. Dental school is 4 years. Following graduation most dentists in New York State complete a one year general residency program. This is usually done in a hospital and is a full time paid position. Some dentists will then pursue further education in specialty areas as I have described in an earlier chapter. At this time dentistry is, in my opinion, an outstanding career if you can afford the education. Tuition averages $40,000 a year. A four year program plus the cost of books and instruments may exceed $200,000. Financing is available but consider the accumulation of debt if you already financed a college education. Certainly the cost of a dental education at a state school is less and is in the range of

$15,000 to $20,000 per year. Gifted students may receive some scholarship money. There may also be programs available from the military to pay some of the tuition in return for the dentist spending a number of years as a military dentist.

Is it worth it? Dentistry still offers the opportunity to run a small to medium sized health care business with relatively little intervention from insurance companies. Insurance companies will dictate fees but only if the dentist chooses to participate in insurance plans. Dental practice offers the opportunity to do very interesting and creative work. This is true for the gifted science student who wants to work for him or herself. Managing a staff, doing marketing and of course doing the various dental procedures is challenging and rewarding. If you want to have immediate gratification then dentistry will offer it. When you see a patient in pain, treat the cause of the pain (endodontic or root canal problem, decayed tooth, gum abscess) and then see immediate relief, you have had a uniquely satisfying experience. The profession is very rewarding financially. Net after tax salaries in the USA average about $200,000 per year for full time dentists in private practice. Of course one may choose to teach and practice part time. There are also careers in the military or in full time education. You may also choose to be an employee in a large practice. This provides an opportunity to provide patient care and not have to manage a business or invest in a facility. The cost of setting up a dental office is about the cost of a nice car per treatment room. Again this can be financed but paying back the debt with interest is costly. So as a patient you should be able to understand that the dentist may be paying back loans for college, dental school, graduate school and the cost of equipment and furnishings for the office. This is in addition to overhead for rent, payroll, insurance and laboratory fees. When a patient is told that the cost of a cap is similar to the cost of an expensive suit remember that the dentist will net only 35% on average after overhead expenses. The dentist will then pay taxes on the net and then use the remaining money to pay for personal expenses including the loans we discussed earlier. For all of these reasons the cost of private dental care is high.

Dental Hygiene training requires a 2 to 3 year program after high school. This is a full time program. Admission is competitive since the number of hygiene schools is few. The training includes extensive academic courses in the biologic sciences and in the manual techniques. Training is followed by a state examination and a license. Hygienists can work full time or part time. Many hygienists choose to work 2 to 3 days a week allowing more time for raising a family. Yes most hygienists are women but of course hygiene school is open to men as well. The salary ranges from $35 to $40 per hour. Full time positions include perks such as vacation, and holiday pay. What do hygienists do? In addition to cleaning teeth they do non surgical periodontal treatment. Hygienists are also licensed to remove decay and place temporary fillings. They may take X-rays. Some hygienists receive additional training and are allowed to administer local anesthesia and nitrous oxide under the direct supervision of the dentist. The other work, such as scaling, prophys and X-rays may be done under indirect supervision meaning the dentist does not need to be in the office but a dentist should be near by to help with patient care if necessary.

The dental assistants' duties include the following: assisting the dentist by passing instruments, sterilizing instruments, taking and developing X-rays, office sanitation and all of the clerical duties ranging from answering the phone to doing insurance forms. They may also teach patients oral hygiene techniques. Salaries range from $7.00 to $20.00 per hour and include benefits for full time assistants such as health insurance, vacation time and pension plans.

The dental technician usually works in a commercial dental laboratory which may employ from 2 to 40 people. The duties range from working with plaster models to creating porcelain restorations (or caps and bridges). Today the fabrication of many restorations is done by computer. This is called cad cam technology. The technician receives prescriptions from the dentist for varies products ranging from dentures to caps and bridges as well as porcelain inlays and onlays. The technician will often communicate directly with the dentist to serve the needs of the patient. The owner of the laboratory must be a certified dental technician. A technician may earn an hourly wage of $10 to $40 dollars per hour or he may own the laboratory and make much more money depending on the size of the laboratory. This could be $200,000 a year or 2 million.

CHAPTER 21

Management of Dental Problems When You Are Away

Typical problems are: a cap falls off, filling breaks, pain with or without infection or swelling. Generally it is best to wait until you return home. **It is a good idea to call your dentist and describe the problem. He may be able to prescribe an antibiotic and pain medication by telephone**. If you and your dentist agree that this should not wait then proceed as follows. If you are in the USA, your dentist may be able to find an appropriate dentist for you. If you cannot reach your dentist consider calling your physician who may be able to help you obtain antibiotics and pain medication. If neither of your doctors is available I suggest calling any local periodontist and asking the periodontist to suggest one of the best dentists available to help you with an emergency. The periodontist may see you if it is the type of dental emergency he can handle.

If you are out of the country you may call the U.S. consulate and ask for a referral.

The emergency room of a major hospital is a possibility. If the hospital has a dental program then a dental resident should be available. Of course have as little permanent treatment done as is appropriate. In most major cities in the USA you will find good dental care. Out of this country you can find good dental care in Israel, Italy, the Scandinavian countries especially Sweden, Canada, South Africa, Germany and the UK. I'm basing this list on publications I have read from these countries. For example Italian and Israeli periodontists have contributed state of the art information on implants and periodontal treatment.

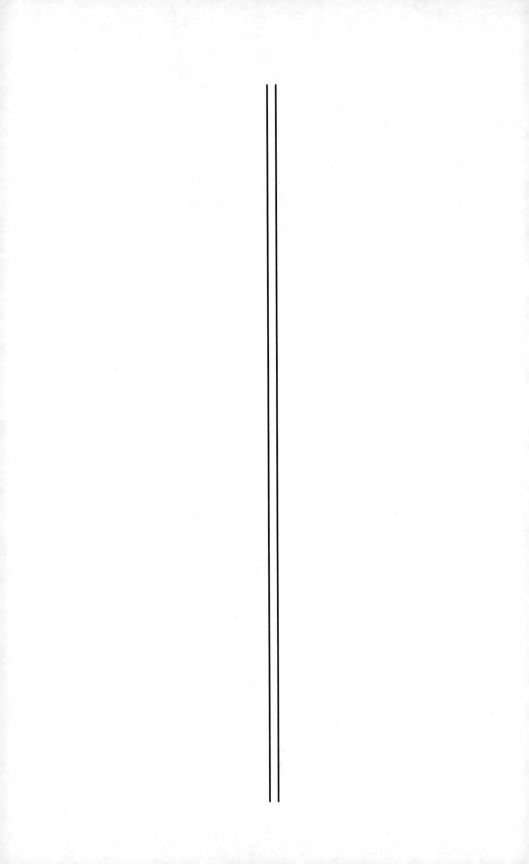

CHAPTER 22	Good Home Remedies for Acute Dental Problems?

Dental problems can happen when you can't contact your dentist. What can you do in the interim? Common problems are: a cap falling off, fillings break, a denture tooth falls off, pain, bleeding gum tissue, swelling or any combination of these events. Many caps that fall off can be temporarily replaced using a denture adhesive as cement. Entire multiunit fixed bridges can fall off and may be simply repositioned without cement until you can see your dentist. Temporary filling materials can be obtained in drug stores. Look in the aisle that has toothpaste and tooth brushes. Use these materials to temporarily cement the cap or bridge. Also use this to cover a broken filling until you can see the dentist. A denture tooth can be recemented with crazy glue.

For pain the best over the counter medication is ibuprofen, up to 800 mg to start, then 2 tabs every 4 hours but do not exceed the recommended dose. If the ibuprofen doesn't work you may add 1000 mg of Tylenol 20 to 30 minutes after taking the ibuprofen. Tylenol comes in 500mg and also 650 mg capsules. These medications are good for a day or two after which the ibuprofen can cause stomach bleeding as does aspirin. After several days Tylenol can cause liver damage. If you are taking Tylenol don't drink alcohol. Alcohol also adversely affects the liver and will potentiate the harmful effects of Tylenol. Ibuprofen can also interfere with the effectiveness of many blood pressure medications. So once again take ibuprofen only if Tylenol is inadequate and for only 24 hours. If you have a narcotic medication remaining from a previous episode you can take it as directed on the label. Again be careful if you are taking other medications that are depressants. Common depressant drugs include Valium, Benadryl, and Xanax. It is a good idea to check with your physician or pharmacist. In fact if you can't contact your dentist, your physician will usually prescribe something appropriate for pain.

If you have swelling and pain you most likely have a dental infection. You can take an antibiotic that you have in the house. If possible consult with your dentist or if he is not available then consult with your physician. If neither your physician nor your dentist is available and you have some remaining penicillin then take one tablet every 4 to 6 hours or 1 tablet 4 times per day. Note the directions prescribed on the bottle. Taking 1 or 2 doses daily won't help. After a few weeks the problem will come back. What other antibiotics are useful for dental infections? In order of effectiveness: Clindamycin, Ciprofoxin, Tetracycline and Erythromycin (Zithromax).

Antibiotics do not cure dental infections. They will help until a dentist can remove the cause.

Be mindful that antibiotics can occasionally have serious side effects. For example the Penicillin family of drugs can cause life threatening allergic reactions. If you take Penicillin and subsequently develop hives and difficulty breathing, call 911 or go to a hospital emergency room immediately. Antibiotics, especially if taken for many days, can cause persistent diarrhea and ulcerative colitis. In some cases a section of the colon will require resection to treat the ulceration. Clindamycin is the most common drug causing this problem. Stop the antibiotic if diarrhea occurs and call your doctor immediately.

Remedies seen in the drug store can be of some help. Liquids containing eugenol can give some temporary relief if placed on a decayed tooth. Of course what you do depends on the type of pain you are having. If you are having pain that is constant and severe, you need immediate attention. Go to the E.R. of your local hospital.

What if you simply have sensitivity to cold affecting one tooth? If the sensitivity disappears seconds after the cold stimulus is removed then you probably have a problem called root sensitivity. This is caused by gum recession secondary to brushing too firmly with a hard brush.

A good temporary solution is the use of Sensodyne toothpaste. Used over a period of days, a chemical in the toothpaste renders the root less sensitive to cold. Obviously you should also avoid cold foods for a while.

Generalized soreness or pain in the mouth with ulcerations is usually secondary to a viral infection. The most common virus involved is the herpes simplex virus. This virus causes cold sores. Denavir is a prescription medication that will make the ulcer resolve more quickly. Abreve is an over the counter medication which also speeds up the healing process. You may buy over the counter solutions or pastes containing Benzocaine for symptomatic relief. A common brand is Xylactin B.

Generalized bleeding from the gum tissue can be treated temporarily with very gentle cleaning and rinsing with a Chlorhexidiene mouth rinse or with Listerine. If you have severe bleeding from a local area such as between two teeth and the bleeding doesn't stop within five minutes, what do you do? Take a small piece of gauze, cotton or even a teabag and place direct pressure on the area. Tea contains tannic acid which is a mild hemostatic agent. The pressure should be maintained for at least 15 minutes. Do not rinse and spit. If you rinse and spit after the bleeding stops you will dislodge the clot that formed and the bleeding will recur. Avoid hot foods and beverages for at least 48 hours and don't chew on the affected area. If you are taking a drug like coumadin and the bleeding recurs several times then consider going to the E.R. of the local hospital for help.

CHAPTER 23	Restorative Dentistry. Should I Have My Teeth Capped?

Teeth need to be restored when part of the tooth structure has been lost due to decay or fracture. The tooth may be restored in different ways depending on the amount of lost tooth structure, as well as the esthetic and biomechanical requirements. A filling is appropriate if a small amount of tooth structure is lost. When most of the tooth structure is lost then a cap, or crown as it is called in the profession, is required due to the mechanical requirements. In other words large fillings fall out or fracture because too little natural tooth structure remains to support and retain the filling material. A crown can replace a large amount of tooth structure. The crown is retained by preparing the remaining tooth with nearly parallel walls of tooth structure so that friction is created when the crown or cap is cemented to the tooth. The cement acts as a seal to prevent the ingress of bacteria around the periphery. The cement also adds to the retention of the crown. Crowns will sometimes fall off because there was too little tooth structure remaining to provide adequate frictional resistance to retain the crown. Fillings will fracture for the same reasons, too little tooth structure remaining or too large a filling.

There are several materials used to fabricate fillings. The common filling materials are: composite resins, glass ionomers, resin ionomers, ceramics (all of the previous four are white fillings), silver amalgam and gold. Gold is being used less frequently because of its higher cost and unacceptable color in our culture. **Silver amalgam is being used less frequently because of the esthetic requirements of some patients and because of concerns regarding the systemic toxicity of mercury in amalgam. The American Dental**

Association has reviewed the available evidence on this issue and has stated that silver amalgam restorations are not a health hazard. Therefore removing silver amalgam fillings and replacing them with white fillings is not required for health reasons. You may find more information on this issue and other dental care issues at www.ada.org which is the website of the American Dental Association. Many patients and dentists now prefer white fillings because of the more natural appearance. In some situations the white filling is more resistant to fracture. Caps or crowns are made from: porcelain (a ceramic material) fused to metal, porcelain alone, composite resins and Zirconium. The type of material used is determined by the esthetic and biomechanical requirements of each situation. The dentist will help you to make the appropriate choice.

Missing teeth can be replaced in several different ways. One or more teeth may be replaced by a fixed prosthesis or bridge supported by teeth. A removable denture may be used to replace several teeth and is supported by attaching clasps to the remaining teeth. A complete denture can be used to replace teeth when all of the natural teeth have been lost. The complete denture is held in by adhesion to the underlying gum tissue. The saliva between the gum tissue and the acrylic denture base creates some retention in the upper arch but less retention is present in the lower arch. Dental implants may be used to support a single crown, many crowns or a full or partial denture. More information is in the chapter on dental implants.

The porcelain veneer or laminate is a unique restoration used to enhance dental esthetics.

The veneer is usually made by the dental technician but can be made by the dentist. Minimal surface preparation of the tooth is followed by bonding of the veneer (as thin as an egg shell) to the facial surface of one or more front teeth. Veneers are used to correct unsightly color and shape problems. Advantages of the veneer compared to a cap are: perfect transmission of light resulting in an excellent esthetic result, minor tooth preparation, and no impingement on the gum tissue. The disadvantages are: fragility and useful only for teeth in good condition except for color or shape issues.

All of the restorations described in the previous paragraphs are provided by the general or restorative dentist. Sometimes a patient with complex restorative needs will be referred to a Prosthodontist who has special training to help satisfy those needs.

Cost is determined by the materials used and the number of teeth being restored. For example a composite filling may cost $400. A ceramic inlay may cost $800. The cost of a cap or crown may be $1000. The charge for fixed bridges is typically $1000 per unit. For example it may be necessary to use 4 natural teeth to support a fixed bridge used to replace 4 missing front teeth. In this case 4 caps and 4 pontics (replaced missing teeth are called pontics), total 8 units and may cost $1000 per unit for a total of $8000. A removable partial denture or full denture may cost $1500. An implant supported restoration, that is the abutment post and cap supported by the implant, may cost $2500 per unit. Porcelain veneers or laminates cost about $1000 per unit.

Typical problems occurring after placement of multiple restorations are: discomfort in a tooth, irritation of the surrounding gum tissue, discomfort when biting and unacceptable esthetics. For these reasons it is a good idea to have large restorations cemented temporarily.

By doing this temporary cementation one can have problems corrected more easily. For example, endodontic treatment can be done without making a hole in the new bridge. A painful gum problem can be corrected easily by removing the bridge and reshaping part of the bridge that may have been impinging on the gum tissue. Esthetic problems can be corrected by returning the bridge to the dental laboratory to change the color of the porcelain. Once the bridge is permanently cemented it cannot be removed without destroying it. After several weeks of symptom free wear the bridge must be permanently cemented to prevent bacteria from causing new decay.

Most general dentists spend most of their office time doing restorative dentistry. If you use the principles I described earlier in this guide to choose a good dentist then it is likely that you will be satisfied with the restorative dentistry provided to you.

Summary

Seeking and maintaining good health is a two way responsibility. As a patient it is your responsibility to find the best practitioner for you. I have attempted to describe how to do that. It is also your responsibility to follow the recommendations of the doctor you choose. It is the duty of the doctor to perform in a way that meets or exceeds the standard of care. As you know there are no guarantees in life. Luck and genetics play a role in health. Unfortunately there are times when even the best doctor and the most compliant patient fail to achieve a good result. We should choose the best treatment plan and the best doctor and give ourselves the opportunity to be successful. Someone said that golf is a parody on life. You can hit a great golf shot but if the ball hits a rock and bounces into the water you will be penalized. It doesn't seem fair but that's golf. However if you keep hitting good golf shots, you will score better than if you hit poor shots. The same is true in life. All we can do is make quality choices and hope for the best.

APPENDIX I
HELPFUL WEBSITES

1. Perio.org: The American Academy of Periodontology, for information about periodontal disease and to find a periodontist

2. Aaoms.org: American Association of Oral and Maxillofacial Surgeons for information about oral surgery

3. Nysdental.org: New York State Dental Association. To find a dentist or for peer review

4. Nassaudental.org: Nassau County Dental Society. To find a dentist or for peer review

5. Nyucd: NYU College of Dentistry for inexpensive dental care by students under supervision.

6. Agd.org: The Academy of General Dentistry, a source of information about dental health and where to find a dentist

7. Dentalemergency.com: phone numbers of dentists on call for dental emergency care

8. www.ada.org: The American Dental Association for information about dental care

9. North Shore University Health System: to find a dentist or physician on line and to reach the dental clinic for inexpensive dental care

10. Drug interaction checker, on line

11. Dentalplans.com: a source for discounted dental treatment.

12. Carecredit.com: interest free financing for dental treatment

Appendix II
Helpful phone numbers

1. American Academy of Periodontology 800 282 4867

2. American Dental Association 800 621 8099

3. Care Credit: to finance dental treatment interest free 800 365 8295

4. Dr. Corsair for answers to questions about implant surgery and Periodontics 516 536 3366

5. New York State Dental Association 800 255 2100

6. Nassau County Dental Society 516 227 1112

BIBLIOGRAPHY

1. www.AmericanCancerSociety.org

2. cdc.gov, Centers for Disease Control and Prevention. Tooth Loss among persons 65 years old and older.

3. Ridker PM, Silvertown JD. Inflamation, C-Reactive Protein, and Atherothrombosis. J Periodontology (Supl.) 2008;79:1544-1551

4. Taylor GW. Bidirectional Interrelation between Diabetes & Periodontal Disease. Annals of Periodontol Dec. 2001;6:880

5. Becker W, Becker B, Berg R. Periodontal Treatment without Maintenance. J Periodontol 1984;55:505

6. N.Y.Times, 11/22/10, "Radiation Worries for Children in the Dental Office

7. Marx R E. Bisphosphonate induced exposed bone of the jaw. J of Oral and Maxillofacial Surgery 2005;63:156

8. Axelsson P. and Lindhe J. The Effects of Controlled Oral Hygiene. Results after 6 years. J Clin. Perio. 1981;8:239

9. Denture Adhesives and Zinc Toxicity. See Glaxo Smith Klein at www.gsk.com

Notes taken when doing your research

1. A list of what you didn't like about your previous dentists

2. A list of the ideal characteristics of a new dentist.

3. The names and phone numbers of new dentists found during your research.

4. A list of the treatment options you have been given and related costs.

5. A list of all medications you are taking and doctors' phone numbers

A List of Questions for Your Dentist at Your Next Visit